How to Get Great Diabetes Care

What you & your doctor can do to improve your medical care— & your life

Irl B. Hirsch, M.D.
University of Washington
School of Medicine

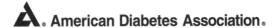

American Diabetes Association

Editorial Director	Peter Banks
Production Director	Carol Segree
Acquisitions Editor	Susan Reynolds
Co-Editors	Sara Henry and Sherrye Landrum
Design and desktop	Insight Graphics
Illustrators	Rebecca Grace Jones and Warren Gebert

American Diabetes Association
1701 North Beauregard Street
Alexandria, VA 22311

Library of Congress Cataloging-in-Publication Data

Hirsch, Irl B. (Irl Bennett), 1958–
    How to get great diabetes care : what you & your doctor can do to improve your medical care—& your life / Irl B. Hirsch.
        p.   cm.
    Includes index.
    ISBN 0-945448-66-X (paper)
    1. Diabetes—Treatment—Standards—United States. I. Title.
RC660.H576   1996
362.1'96462—dc20   96-32863
                                                          CIP

Printed in the United States of America

3 5 7 9 10 8 6 4 2

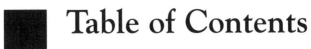

Table of Contents

■ Preface

*"The care of the future should
be the standards of the present."*

In the May 1989 issue of *Diabetes Care*, the American Diabetes Association (ADA) published a position statement entitled "Standards of Medical Care for Patients With Diabetes Mellitus." This document, reviewed by dozens of experts, set guidelines for the treatment of diabetes and its complications. Due to further developments and advances in the field, these Standards of Care were revised in 1994 and, no doubt, will be updated in the future to keep pace with research findings.

An editorial by David C. Robbins, MD, in the same issue described the document as a "Bill of Rights...of the patient with diabetes mellitus." Dr. Robbins suggested that these guidelines be required reading for any professional who deals with diabetic patients, because they are a "valuable model" for health care professionals to "improve their own clinical practice."

Seven years after the first publication of the ADA Standards of Care, doctors need to examine how they are doing both following these guidelines and treating patients with diabetes in general. The results of surveys that have tried to answer this have been disappointing. In general, clinical practice patterns lag far behind advances in medical therapies. This is true for many diseases, such as peptic ulcer disease, congestive heart failure, osteoporosis, and certainly, diabetes. This means that we need to increase our efforts to educate health care professionals. Clinical research continues to provide us with better tools to treat diabetes and its complications. ADA supports and provides professional education as one of its fundamental missions.

People with diabetes have a need to know about the latest developments in diabetic care, says Dr. Robbins in his editorial. "The educated and assertive patient who demands excellence is far more likely to receive it." This book was written with Dr. Robbins' comments in mind. Most of the topics are addressed in enough detail that you will feel comfortable discussing the ADA Standards of Care with your health team members.

One of the most fascinating aspects of clinical medicine is that new research findings can dramatically change what we do in practice. These changes can be so abrupt that news of them does not reach the medical literature or lay press immediately. The treatment of stomach ulcers with antibiotics is one example of this. So, if the treatment your doctor recommends is not covered in the Standards, ask about it. It may be based on new research that has not yet been included in the Standards of Care.

In each chapter a major topic reviewed in the Standards of Care is described. This book may be used as a reference if you have a particular question, such as "what are the recommended cholesterol or blood pressure levels for someone with diabetes?" Or it may be used as a guide to help you measure the care you are getting. It is my sincere hope that the pages that follow will help you become more knowledgeable about diabetes, and that this will help you participate in and receive better health care.

Irl B. Hirsch

Acknowledgments

This book would not have been possible without the support of many people. I thank all of the staff at the University of Washington Diabetes Care Center for assistance in our mission to improve the lives of people with diabetes. In particular, I thank Dr. Jerry P. Palmer for trusting my vision to accomplish our goals. I also thank Drs. Jay S. Skyler, Philip E. Cryer, Julio V. Santiago, David E. Goldstein, and Patrick J. Boyle, who taught me how to be a better physician able to treat such a complicated condition. This book would not have been possible without my patients and their families, who, as a group, taught me the most about the management of diabetes.

I thank Sherry Dodson, Lori Hall, and Lisa Oberg, who all helped me gather important information included in this book. I appreciate the guidance and encouragement of Susan Reynolds from the American Diabetes Association.

Writing this book has been an enjoyable but challenging task. I am grateful to my wife, Ruth, and my daughter, Barbara, for their support and encouragement throughout this project.

Finally, a word of appreciation to my parents for their support and love.

■ 1

The Path to Great Care

You may have just been diagnosed with diabetes, or you may have had it for years. In either case, it's time to get involved in your medical care. To get great care you have to play the starring role—the patient who is also number one on the health care team. Diabetes is a complicated condition. You, your doctor, and other members of your health care team must work together so you will feel your best each day and prevent or postpone complications. This book is the tool to help you get the best possible care for your diabetes.

The Standards of Care

In 1989 the American Diabetes Association (ADA) published the "Standards of Medical Care for Patients With Diabetes Mellitus" (called simply Standards of Care). The Standards of Care tells doctors and patients what they need to do for "state-of-the-art" diabetes therapy. It was updated in 1994 and will be updated again when new research suggests even better treatments for diabetes. The Standards of Care gives you target levels for your blood glucose, blood pressure, and lipids; the tests to screen for diabetes complications; and things to discuss at each visit with your doctor. The Standards of Care is one of 21 position statements published by the ADA.

The 21 position statements spell out what is required to treat diabetes. Most people with diabetes do not now receive this level of care. Research has shown that if you do, you are less likely to develop complications and more likely to live a healthier life. Many doctors may not have heard about the Standards of Care or the position statements. If you and your doctor work together to follow these guidelines, your health will benefit greatly.

The position statements contain everything from foot care guidelines and nutrition recommendations to hospital admission guidelines. They're published in ADA journals and are approved by several committees. Position statements are reviewed each year and updated when necessary.

A *technical review* is a study of all the scientific writings and research about a topic related to diabetes. This review often supports a position statement. A *consensus statement*—also published by ADA—is the opinion of a panel of experts about a medical issue related to diabetes. The consensus statement, unlike the position statement, is not reviewed and isn't an official ADA opinion.

All of the latest position statements and consensus statements are published each year in a supplement to *Diabetes Care*, one of the ADA journals for health care providers.

Self-Monitoring of Blood Glucose

You eat food for energy and growth. Your body turns the food into glucose (sugar). Glucose travels around your body in the blood. The glucose has to get into the cells before it can be used for energy. If you have insulin-dependent (type I) diabetes, your body does not produce insulin, the hormone that helps glucose get into cells. If you have non-insulin-dependent (type II) diabetes, either you don't make enough insulin or it doesn't work well. With either type of diabetes, you can't use the glucose, and it builds up in your blood. You can learn to control your blood glucose levels with careful meal planning, exercise, and insulin or oral medication if you need it. But first you need to know where your blood glucose level is.

No development since insulin has been as important as the ability to check your blood glucose level at home. In the past, the only way to check your blood glucose at home was with urine glucose testing. This was an awkward and not very dependable method. Reports from 1978 show that self-monitoring of blood glucose (SMBG) dramatically improves a person's diabetes control because it gives you important information needed to make adjustments in insulin, food, and exercise. Since the early 1980s, the meters have gotten smaller, more accurate, and easier to use.

You need to be taught how to check your own blood glucose by a diabetes educator, and you need to review the procedure with your health care team from time to time. That is when you'll hear about new developments that make it more accurate and easier to do. Discuss with your doctor how many times a day and when you should check your blood glucose. There are a lot of different types of blood glucose meters, and your doctor or diabetes educator can help you decide which one is right for you.

More Advances in Treatment

In the 1980s, another tool was developed to help you check your blood glucose levels. This blood test measures your average blood glucose levels for the past 3–4 months. That's why it doesn't matter what time of day you have the test or what you've eaten before you have it. A glycated hemoglobin (HbA_{1c}) test measures the amount of glucose that has joined with the hemoglobin (red blood cells) in your blood. The more glucose there is in your blood, the more hemoglobin will join with it. Once joined, the cells stay that way for the life of the cell—about 120 days. The glycated hemoglobin number gives you and your doctor a measurement of your day to day diabetes control

---

The History of Diabetes Treatment

Although diabetes has been known as a disease for 2,000 years, it is only in the last 100 years that we've been able to treat it. At the turn of the century, a patient with type I diabetes lived less than 1 year from diagnosis. Before the discovery of insulin in 1921, it was found that patients with insulin-dependent diabetes could live longer (weeks or months) by drastically cutting back on the food they ate—less than 500 calories per day, with some days of total fasting. (It was difficult to get patients to go along with this, however.)

History, *continued*

Fortunately, in the summer of 1921, at the University of Toronto, experiments directed by Dr. Frederick Banting, a young surgeon, and Charles Best, a fourth-year physiology student, resulted in the discovery of insulin. These studies took place in the laboratory of J.J.R. Macleod and with the assistance of J.B. Collip, a biochemist. (You may want to read about this in *The Discovery of Insulin*, by Michael Bliss—fascinating reading.) In 1923, Banting and Macleod received the Nobel prize for medicine for discovering insulin.

People quickly realized that insulin was not a cure for diabetes. And although it helped keep people alive, it created several other problems. The injections had to be continued for the rest of the patient's life. The insulin acted quickly, so injections had to be given often. There was no way to guarantee the potency of the insulin, so decisions about what dose to use were difficult. Doctors in the 1920s also disagreed about what level of blood glucose control was best—a debate that went on for many years. If patients took enough insulin to prevent glucose from showing up in the urine, they might have very low blood glucose (hypoglycemia), which could even be fatal. In these early days, people ignored diet or exercise, believing that the insulin could solve all of their problems. These ideas have changed over the years. In the 1930s and 1940s, longer-acting insulins were created.

These insulins were developed for convenience. NPH, lente, ultra-lente, and protomine zinc insulins allowed patients with type I diabetes to get by with only one injection daily. This practice continues today, but few patients with type I diabetes can maintain normal or near-normal blood glucose on this treatment. Of course, until recently, we had no proof that maintaining "tight" blood glucose is important for type I diabetes. On the other hand, many patients with type II diabetes who take insulin can get excellent blood glucose control with only one daily injection.

over a 3–4 month period. Other names for glycated hemo-globin are glycohemoglobin and glycosylated hemoglobin.

The team approach for managing diabetes was first intro-duced in the early 1980s. Rather than just seeing a doctor, people with diabetes began to work with a team made up of a doctor, nurse, registered dietitian (RD), psychologist, social worker, and pharmacist. These people became dia-betes educators. A national organization, the American Association of Diabetes Educators (AADE), was set up in 1973, and the first exam for the certification of diabetes educators (CDE) was in 1986.

These three—self blood glucose testing, the glycated hemoglobin test, and the health care team—made it pos-sible for us to research whether good diabetes control can prevent diabetes complications. Before these develop-ments, there was great debate as to whether good diabetes control was important.

The question of how important blood glucose control is in preventing complications was answered (at least for peo-ple with type I diabetes) with the results of the Diabetes Control and Complications Trial (DCCT). This was a 9.5-year-long study reported in 1993, and the results were dra-matically clear. People who keep their blood glucose closer to normal levels with tight control can prevent or delay 50–60 percent of the complications caused by diabetes.

Another study, also published in 1993, the Stockholm Diabetes Intervention Study agreed with the DCCT. Blood glucose levels that are kept near normal with intensive dia-betes therapy can cut down on diabetic retinopathy (eye disease), nephropathy (kidney disease), and neuropathy (nerve disease).

Studies show that people with type II diabetes probably gain the same benefits from having near normal glucose levels, particularly with regard to their eyes, kidneys, and nerves. This topic is discussed in greater detail in Chapter 3.

Diseases Linked to Diabetes

Diabetes can lead to other serious ailments. You need to know what can go wrong so you can work with your doctor to prevent it. Control of your blood glucose levels and proper treatment can prevent or slow down many diseases. Here's a brief rundown.

Eye diseases

The retina is like a "movie screen" in the back of your eyes that receives images. Retinopathy is a disease of the small vessels that supply the retina with blood. When caught early, this disease can be slowed or stopped. In *nonproliferative retinopathy*, the little blood vessels may close up or leak blood into the eyes, and this causes blurry vision. *Proliferative retinopathy* is more serious but less likely to happen. Many new blood vessels grow in the retina but break easily. Blood may leak and interfere with your sight. Also, scar tissue may form on the retina and damage your vision. (See Chapter 7.)

Kidney problems (nephropathy)

Normally, blood is cleaned in your kidneys as it passes through small blood vessels. High blood glucose causes the kidneys to filter the blood more often. In nephropathy, these overworked blood vessels become blocked and leak. They can't filter well, blood pressure rises, and protein is allowed to slip through into your urine. A protein called albumin is one that slips through. *Microalbuminuria*, which means very small amounts of albumin in your urine, is the first sign of diabetic kidney disease. It is also a sign of your increased risk for heart attack. (See Chapter 8.)

Nerve damage (neuropathy)

Too much blood glucose damages the nervous system. Damaged nerves either don't send messages, send them too slowly, or send them at the wrong time. This can cause many different health problems, such as numbness or burning in your feet, and can contribute to infections in your limbs. (See Chapter 11.)

High blood pressure (hypertension)

High blood pressure can lead to heart attack, circulation problems, and stroke and increase your risk of eye disease and diabetic nephropathy. (See Chapter 9.)

Whether you have type I or type II diabetes, it is to your benefit to work on keeping your blood glucose near normal levels and to see your doctor regularly for help reaching your goals. This book explains each of the standards for diabetes care and why they are important to you. Armed with this up-to-date information, you and your health care team can design a thorough diabetes care game plan that is uniquely suited to you and your needs.

■ 2

Screening for Diabetes

Many people have diabetes without being aware of it—as many as 7 million diabetic Americans have not yet been diagnosed. A way to help determine whether a person has diabetes or may develop it is to look for certain risk factors. The three major risk factors are having family members with diabetes, being overweight, and belonging to an ethnic group that has a higher-than-average risk. A fourth risk factor is being older than 45 and having any of the other three risk factors.

Identifying whether you have these risk factors helps doctors diagnose diabetes as early as possible. When you catch diabetes early, you have a better chance of avoiding complications down the line. Doctors do not run blood tests to check for diabetes on every patient, and they take risk factors as well as symptoms into account when deciding to test. On average, people have type II diabetes for 10 years before they know they have it. And complications are often the reason it is finally discovered. If you have risk factors for diabetes but do not yet have it, you can improve your chances of not getting it by changing what you eat, beginning to exercise, and/or losing some weight.

Risk Factors You Can't Change

Family history of diabetes

If your mother, father, brother, or sister has diabetes, your risk of developing it is higher than if you have an aunt, uncle, or grandparent with diabetes. A 1976–1980 survey of people aged 20–54 years with type II diabetes showed that nearly half of them had a parent with diabetes and more than a third had a brother or sister with diabetes.

Type II diabetes is more closely linked to genetics, but there is also a genetic link with type I diabetes. If you have a parent or brother or sister with type I diabetes, you have only a 3–5 percent chance of also developing it. This risk is higher than for the general population—the risk for a school-age child in the general population is 0.3 percent— but it is not a huge risk. However, if your identical twin has type I diabetes, you have a 35–40 percent risk of also developing it.

The problem is that, even today, many people have diabetes and do not know it. There's always a chance your relatives may have diabetes and simply have not been diagnosed.

It's also important to remember that, although type I diabetes usually develops before age 30, it can develop at any age.

Race

Certain minorities, including American Indians, Hispanics, and African Americans, are at a higher risk for developing type II diabetes. Many of these ethnic groups were historically hunters or farmers who went long periods without food and tended to be lean. Today most people have plenty to eat but get little exercise. Many people have become obese and developed diabetes and high blood pressure. The very trait that helped them to survive periods of feast and famine now puts them at risk.

African Americans. After age 45, diabetes in black people is 1.4–2.3 times as frequent as in white people. The frequency of diabetes in black Americans has been increasing faster than in white Americans. From 1963 to 1985, the rate of diabetes doubled for white people but tripled for black people. Diabetes was particularly more common in black women. One study of 11,100 people showed diabetes in 15 percent of black women, 11 percent of black men, 7 percent of white women, and 7 percent of white men.

Hispanic Americans. Hispanics, particularly Mexican Americans, are also at higher risk for developing type II diabetes. Mexican Americans have two to three times higher risk of developing diabetes compared with non-Hispanics. The risk is especially high for women.

Asian Americans. Asians (Chinese, Filipino, Japanese, Asian Indian, Korean, and Vietnamese) and Pacific Islanders (Hawaiian, Samoan, and Guamanian) also have a higher risk. For example, for second-generation Japanese Americans (people whose parents moved here from Japan), type II diabetes occurs in 20 percent of men and 16 percent of women.

American Indians. Diabetes is also more common in North American Indians and Alaska Natives. A 1987 survey found that 12.2 percent of American Indians had diabetes, compared to 5.2 percent in the general population.

History of diabetes during pregnancy

Diabetes during pregnancy, *gestational diabetes*, occurs in about 3 percent of all pregnancies, and usually disappears after the baby is born. Women who have had gestational diabetes, however, are at a higher risk of developing diabetes later in life. Nearly 40 percent of women who have had diabetes during pregnancy develop type II diabetes within 20 years of their pregnancies. Because the symptoms are mild, this form of diabetes may not be diagnosed. High blood glucose levels in mothers can increase the chances of problems with the baby, so it's important that pregnant women maintain normal blood glucose levels. All women should be checked for gestational diabetes during the second trimester of pregnancy. Women with diabetes during pregnancy tend to have babies weighing more than 9 pounds. If you have had a large baby, you'll be considered at higher risk for developing gestational diabetes in any later pregnancies, as well as for developing type II diabetes later in life.

Risk Factors You May Be Able to Change

Impaired glucose tolerance

Impaired glucose tolerance means that your blood glucose level (the amount of sugar in your blood) is not normal, but you don't have diabetes. Having impaired glucose tolerance means you have a higher risk of developing type II diabetes. Of 1,000 people with impaired glucose tolerance, 10–50 will develop diabetes, while the risk for the general population is only 2.5 people out of 1,000.

If your doctor suspects impaired glucose tolerance, you will have to take an oral glucose tolerance test. You cannot eat for 10 hours before this test (usually overnight), and then you are given a sugary drink containing 75 grams of glucose. You will have your blood drawn every 30 minutes over a 2-hour period; the blood is sent to a laboratory to be analyzed. You have impaired glucose intolerance if
- your blood glucose levels at the beginning of the test are below 140 mg/dl
- the 2-hour blood glucose levels are 140–200 mg/dl
- at least one other blood glucose has a level higher than 200 mg/dl

If the 2-hour level is greater than 200 mg/dl (with one other blood glucose above 200 mg/dl and the initial level less than 140 mg/dl), you have diabetes.

If you have impaired glucose tolerance, you won't develop the eye, kidney, and nerve disease linked with diabetes, but you are at a higher risk for developing heart disease and stroke. Your doctor will probably suggest that you do whatever you can to lower your risks for developing both heart disease and diabetes. You can do this by planning your meals and increasing the amount you exercise. These steps will help you lose weight and lower the amount of cholesterol in your blood and your blood pressure.

Certain drugs can cause impaired glucose tolerance or even diabetes. If you have any other risk factors for type II diabetes, only use these drugs with caution. *Ask your doctor if he or she should substitute other drugs or treatments, considering your risk factors for developing diabetes.* These types of drugs include steroids such as prednisone and dexamethasone, furosemide (Lasix), thiazide diuretics such as hydrochlorothiazide (Diurel), ß-blockers such as propranolol (Inderal), and niacin (Nicobid and Nicolar). Table 2–1 provides a more complete list.

High blood pressure or high blood fat

If you have either high blood pressure or high levels of blood fats called lipids (these include cholesterol and triglycerides), you're considered at higher risk for developing diabetes. In Chapters 9 and 10, you'll find a detailed discussion of blood pressure and lipids.

Overweight

Perhaps the most important risk factor that you can do something about is obesity. Weight loss can be difficult, because of the lifestyle changes involved and because you may be genetically disposed to be heavy. Some people may need to build a daily exercise routine into a sedentary lifestyle and overhaul cooking and eating habits. Exercise makes you healthier even if you are still overweight.

Check out your weight. You're considered obese if your weight is more than 20 percent over your ideal body weight. There are several ways to determine your ideal body weight. One way is to compare your weight to a chart

Table 2-1
Drugs That May Raise Blood Glucose Levels

Class of Drug	Example
Steroids	Prednisone (Deltazone)
	Dexamethasone (Decadron)*
Sex steroids	Testosterone (Virilon, Testaderm, Androderm)*
	Progesterone (Provera)
Diuretics	Hydrochlorothiazide (Hydrodiuril and others)
	Furosemide (Lasix)
ß-Blockers	Propranolol (Inderal)
	Atenolol (Tenormin)
	Metoprolol (Lopressor and Toprol)
Lipid lowering	Niacin (Nicobid and Nicolar)
Antibiotics	Isoniazid (INH)
	Pentamidine (Pentam)**
Immunosuppressive	Cyclosporin (Sandimmune)
Thyroid hormone	Levothyroxine (Synthroid, Levothroid, and others)*
Other hormones	Megestrol (Megace)
	Octreotide (Sandostatin)**

* when used in high doses
** may cause hypoglycemia or hyperglycemia

of acceptable weights. (See Table 2–2.) This will give you a range of weights for your height.

Consider your BMI. Another way to determine whether you are obese is to look at your body mass index, or BMI.

To calculate this, multiply your weight by 705. Divide this answer by your height in inches. Now divide by your height again. The answer is your BMI. Compare it to the figures below:

20–25: normal weight
25–30: overweight
30+: severely overweight

Your BMI will give you a better idea of whether you are overweight than whether you've gained weight recently. If you weigh 15 pounds more now than you did a decade ago, but your BMI is 24, you are not considered obese— even though you might really like to lose 10 pounds!

Where do you carry your weight? Where you carry the extra weight also matters. People who have what is called central obesity (shaped like an apple) seem to have a higher risk for developing diabetes than those with peripheral obesity (shaped like a pear, carrying the extra weight down low). There is some evidence that black people have a greater tendency to store fat centrally, which may partially explain their higher risk of developing type II diabetes.

Researchers have determined that having fat within your abdomen (called intra-abdominal fat) is even more significant. This fat can be measured with sophisticated X rays and may be higher than normal even if you have a BMI within the normal range, and you don't have obvious central obesity. Having extra intra-abdominal fat apparently increases the risk of both type II diabetes and heart disease.

Table 2–2
Suggested Adult Weight for Men and Women

Height without shoes	Weight without clothes (pounds)
4'10"	91–119
4'11"	94–123
5'0"	97–128
5'2"	104–137
5'3"	107–141
5'4"	111–146
5'5"	114–150
5'6"	118–155
5'7"	121–160
5'8"	125–164
5'9"	129–169
5'10"	132–174
5'11"	136–179
6'0"	140–184
6'1"	144–189
6'2"	148–195
6'3"	152–200
6'4"	156–205
6'5"	160–211
6'6"	164–216

Source: U.S. Department of Agriculture, December 1995.

What the Results Mean to You and Your Doctor

It is not possible to screen everyone or even everyone who has one risk factor for diabetes. At least 78 percent of adults in the United States have one or more of the risk factors noted above, and 23 percent have three or more.

A major goal of a community screening program is to identify who is at risk of developing diabetes. ADA recommends that people with one or more risk factors go to a doctor for evaluation and possible testing. Screening by measuring blood glucose levels with a plasma glucose test—preferably after not eating for 8 hours—should be done only on people with at least one risk factor for having diabetes and pregnant women between the 24th and 28th

---

Questions to Ask Your Doctor

I don't have all the symptoms of diabetes, so how could I have diabetes?

How often should I be tested? What kind of tests?

If I'm diabetic, does that mean that my children will be?

Will I become diabetic when I get pregnant? How will I know?

Questions Your Doctor May Ask You

Does anyone in your family have diabetes? Who?

Does anyone in your family have eye disease, kidney disease, or nerve damage (complications of diabetes)?

What is your ethnic background?

How much did your babies weigh at birth?

Have you ever had a blood glucose test? A glucose tolerance test?

Do you have results of any blood fat (lipid) tests?

Have you ever had protein in your urine?

Are you on any medications?

Are you often thirsty?

Do you urinate frequently? Do you get up at night to urinate?

---

weeks of pregnancy. Testing is also recommended for anyone with a disease that can be a complication of diabetes,
such as various eye diseases or kidney disease, or with any
of the classic symptoms of diabetes, such as excessive thirst
and urination. To diagnose diabetes, an oral glucose tolerance test is needed.

Although the criteria for testing for diabetes will continue
to change, people who have at least one of the risk factors
listed in this chapter and a fasting blood glucose level
below 115 mg/dl should be retested in 3 years. If the fasting blood glucose is above 115 mg/dl but below 126 mg/dl,
your doctor may recommend a glucose tolerance test. If the
fasting blood glucose is above 126 mg/dl, your doctor
should repeat the test, and if the results are again above
126 mg/dl, you will be diagnosed with diabetes.

■ 3

Blood Glucose Control

One of the major problems of diabetes—especially type I diabetes—is that it can lead to other health problems, including eye disease, kidney problems, and nerve damage. Many health care professionals have long believed that carefully controlling the levels of glucose in your blood may help prevent or slow the development of these problems. Until recently, we had no proof of this.

An important study completed in 1993 resolved the debate for people with type I diabetes. The DCCT lasted for nearly 10 years and studied 1,441 people. The people who participated in this trial received either standard treatment, much like most people with diabetes receive, or intensified treatment. The standard treatment was one or two insulin injections daily, occasional home blood glucose tests, and information about diet and exercise. The people in the intensive program took three or more daily injections (or used an insulin infusion pump), tested their blood glucose at least four times a day, and paid careful attention to meal planning and exercise. The goal of this group was to have normal or near normal levels of blood glucose.

What Happens With Close Control of Glucose Levels?

Benefits

The results of the trial were dramatic. The people who followed the intensive therapy—with frequent blood glucose checks and three or more injections a day—had significantly fewer cases of eye and kidney disease caused by diabetes. The first appearance of the eye disease retinopathy was reduced by 27 percent, and the appearance of more advanced retinopathy was reduced by 34–76 percent. Proliferative retinopathy, the severe type that damages your vision, and laser therapy to treat it were reduced by 45 percent. Most impressive, retinopathy got worse as glycated hemoglobin increased. (This shows that any improvement in diabetes control will slow diabetic retinopathy and help you keep it from getting worse.)

In the intensive treatment group, the appearance of the earliest stages of kidney disease (microalbuminuria) was reduced by more than 35 percent, while more advanced kidney disease was reduced by more than 50 percent. Symptoms of nerve damage, called neuropathy, were reduced by 60 percent.

Problems

The major drawback of intensive therapy was severe hypoglycemia, or low blood glucose, which occurred three times more often in the intensive treatment group. (*Severe* means that another person was needed to help treat the

The Diabetes Control and Complications Trial (DCCT)

The DCCT was a study of 1,441 people that lasted almost 10 years. In this trial, people with type I diabetes received either conventional therapy or intensive therapy. Conventional therapy was like the standard diabetes care most people receive. They injected insulin once or twice daily (intermediate- and rapid-acting insulin), tested their own blood glucose levels occasionally (at the beginning of the study, only urine glucose testing was done), and received education about diet and exercise. They did not take supplemental insulin based on glucose monitoring.

The primary goals were to avoid symptoms of high blood glucose, such as frequent urination and thirst, frequent low blood glucose, or ketones in the urine. (Ketones are a by-product of fat breakdown that appear when you do not have enough insulin.) Women who became pregnant or were planning a pregnancy received intensive therapy until the time of delivery and then went back to conventional therapy.

Intensive therapy was designed to keep blood glucose levels close to normal by at least three injections of insulin daily or by an insulin infusion pump. People could switch back and forth from multiple injections to a pump if desired. Insulin doses were adjusted daily based on four or more daily home blood glucose measurements, what was eaten, and the amount of exercise scheduled. The blood glucose goals were: before meals 70–120 mg/dl; after meals less than 180 mg/dl; at least one weekly 3 AM measurement greater than 65 mg/dl. The goal for glycated hemoglobin was less than 6.05 percent (the upper limit of the normal range).

DCCT, *continued*

Fewer than 5 percent of people in the intensive therapy group could maintain a normal glycated hemoglobin level—which shows that blood glucose levels through the days were normal. But 44 percent of this group achieved this goal at least once. For the intensive therapy group as a whole, the average glycated hemoglobin level was 7.2 percent. Compare this to 8.9 percent for the conventional therapy group. Blood glucose profiles (people measured their blood glucose seven times in a day) revealed average values of 155 mg/dl for the intensive group and 231 mg/dl for the conventional group.

---

hypoglycemia.) The other major concern was weight gain. People in the intensive therapy group gained about 10 more pounds than people in the other group. This is probably because good control means glucose gets into the cells instead of being lost in the urine.

For People With Type II Diabetes

Now the question arises: What does all this mean for people with type II diabetes? Research up to now supports the same connection between long-term high blood glucose and complications such as eye, nerve, and kidney problems in people with type II diabetes. It appears that how much high blood glucose, not the type of diabetes, best predicts whether these complications will develop. For example, in a 10-year survey of diabetes-related complications in southern Wisconsin, complications from diabetes were linked to high glycated hemoglobin levels. The higher the glycated hemoglobin, the greater the risk for complications.

In 1995, a group from Kimumoto, Japan, reported on a 6-year study similar to the DCCT, with an intensive therapy and a conventional therapy group, for people with type II diabetes. As happened in the DCCT, retinopathy, neuropathy, and nephropathy were all more common in the people on conventional therapy. However, in the Japanese study, the people were thin and had normal cholesterol and triglyceride levels, which is different from most people with type II diabetes in the United States. Still, most scientists believe that excellent blood glucose control with type II diabetes will prevent or delay complications, especially retinopathy, nephropathy, and neuropathy.

Most doctors feel that people with type II diabetes should try to get good blood glucose control with meal planning and exercise alone. People can go a long time without medication, depending on how well they follow their meal plan and exercise routine and how far the diabetes has progressed. However, after awhile, many people need medication to get the same level of glucose control. Early data from a large British study reported that 83 percent of newly diagnosed people with type II diabetes using diet alone require drug therapy within 1 year.

The question about whether to try for normal blood glucose levels arises when people with type II diabetes have to take insulin. Obese people with type II diabetes gain even more weight when started on insulin. After using insulin for 3–12 months, they gain an average of 13 pounds. Improved diabetes control with the addition of a sulfonylurea may also cause weight gain. How do we balance the gain in weight and its effects on the body with the slowing down of complications like retinopathy?

There are also a variety of psychological benefits to improved diabetes control—better quality of life and a sense of well-being. You may feel that you are in control of your diabetes, instead of having it control you. And that is very important.

Who May Not Be Able to Try This

Intensive blood glucose control won't work for everyone. You need to discuss what blood glucose levels are best for you with your doctor. For some people, the risks of the intensive program may outweigh the benefits.

Hypoglycemia

One problem is that some people with diabetes do not know when they are hypoglycemic. Unless they measure their blood glucose frequently, these people may have repeated severe hypoglycemia. For them, trying to maintain normal or near-normal levels of blood glucose can be dangerous or even life threatening because their blood glucose goes too low. These people need to raise their blood glucose targets. If you have had an episode of severe hypoglycemia or are unable to recognize symptoms when your blood glucose drops below 60 mg/dl, ask your doctor what your blood glucose targets should be.

Severe complications

The DCCT study group also warned that people with advanced complications such as the last stages of kidney disease or heart disease should not follow the intensive regimen. The risks are too great. Improved blood glucose control does not appear to help with advanced kidney disease or advanced retinopathy. Bouts of severe hypoglycemia might be too risky for people with serious heart disease because it might prevent the heart from receiving enough oxygen, which could lead to a heart attack.

You may still want to work toward some improvement in your blood glucose control, because it may protect you from other complications. For instance, if you have advanced retinopathy, improving your blood glucose control will not help protect your eyes, but it may help prevent or slow nerve damage due to your diabetes.

Age

You may not want to try intensive therapy for children under age 13. Children below this age were not included in the study, and the evidence suggests that diabetes in the years before puberty may not contribute as much to developing complications as in the years after puberty. Also, hypoglycemia in youngsters—particularly toddlers and infants—may result in brain damage. The risk of hypoglycemia with intensive therapy is not worth it for children. Around the time of puberty, however, most children may benefit from intensive therapy. (The people in the DCCT ranged in age from 13 to 39 years.)

Intensive therapy is usually not recommended for elderly people, because severe hypoglycemia could have more devastating consequences (such as causing a heart attack or stroke) than it would for younger adults.

Life expectancy

If a person has another serious disease, trying for near-normal blood glucose targets may not be recommended.

For example, people with another disease that will shorten life expectancy—such as terminal cancer or AIDS—don't need to try for these goals. It is probably not worth the risk and trouble to get good glucose control because the benefits of it are not realized for years.

Heart disease and stroke
Other reasons not to strive for these goals include advanced heart disease or history of stroke. Hypoglycemia, because it causes an increase in adrenaline (epinephrine) levels, may cause narrowing of the blood vessels that lead to the heart or brain. This in turn can lead to another heart attack or stroke.

Severe hypoglycemia
Also mentioned earlier is the risk of severe low blood glucose or hypoglycemia. People with hypoglycemia unawareness must balance the benefits of good control against the life-threatening risk of severe hypoglycemia.

Recommendations

The DCCT recommended that most people with type I diabetes be treated with intensive therapy with the goal of blood glucose levels "as close to the normal range as safely possible." Because of the problems with hypoglycemia, ADA recommends increasing the blood glucose targets. The study targets were 70–120 mg/dl before meals and at bedtime and less than 180 mg/dl 1.5–2 hours after meals. ADA suggests raising the targets to 80–120 mg/dl before meals and 100–140 mg/dl at bedtime. You and your doctor need to fit the blood glucose goals to your needs, however, especially if you are older.

ADA also recommends the following at the start of intensive therapy:

- frequent blood glucose monitoring (3–4 times a day)
- nutrition counseling
- training in self-management and problem solving
- possible hospitalization for guidance when the therapy is started

What is the bottom line? In the 1994 Standards of Care, ADA gave specific goals of blood glucose therapy for people with diabetes (see Table 3–1). There was no difference between the two major types of diabetes, but blood glucose goals may not be as tight for older people. Pregnant women will have different blood glucose and glycated hemoglobin targets, which are outlined in Chapter 6.

If your doctor does not know about intensive therapy, ADA recommends that you see a diabetes care team to learn about the therapy and for assistance as you go along. Treatment for people with type II diabetes needs to focus on meal planning and exercise with a goal of losing weight. If this therapy does not result in good blood glucose control, glucose-lowering agents and/or insulin may need to be added (see Appendix 1).

You may act immediately after you check your blood glucose or after you have noted a pattern. For example, if a man with type I diabetes wakes up every morning with blood glucose levels above 140 mg/dl, this suggests not only that he needs more insulin right then, but also that some change in his insulin or diet is required the night before. If a woman with type II diabetes taking sulfonylurea and insulin has bedtime blood glucose levels consistently

Table 3–1
Suggested Glycemic Control
(Check with your Doctor)

Test	Nondiabetic	Goal	Action Suggested* If:
Blood glucose before meal	<110	80–120	<80 or >200
Blood glucose at bedtime (mg/dl)	<120	200	<100 or >160
Glycated hemo-globin (%)	<6	<7	>8

* "Action suggested" means that if you fall in this range, you need to make an adjustment of diet, exercise, or medication to bring your blood glucose level back into target range.

learn about the therapy and for assistance as you go along. Treatment for people with type 2 diabetes needs to focus on meal planning and exercise with a goal of losing weight. If this therapy does not result in good blood glucose control, glucose-lowering agents and/or insulin may need to be added (see Appendix 1).

You may act immediately after you check your blood glucose or after you have noted a pattern. For example, if a man with type 1 diabetes wakes up every morning with blood glucose levels above 140 mg/dl, this suggests not only that he needs more insulin right then, but also that

Questions to Ask Your Doctor

Am I a candidate for intensive therapy? If not, why not?

Will you refer me to a dietitian or someone who will help me with an exercise regimen? Does my insurance cover this?

Will you refer me to a certified nurse educator (CDE) to teach me SMBG and how to change my medication based on my blood glucose levels?

What should my blood glucose levels be before meals? After meals? At bedtime?

Can you refer me to an endocrinologist or someone experienced in intensive therapy?

Questions Your Doctor May Ask You

How old are you?

When were you diagnosed with diabetes?

Do you have severe hypoglycemia? hypoglycemia unawareness?

Have you ever passed out because of hypoglycemia?

Do you have heart disease?

Do you have advanced kidney disease (nephropathy)?

Have you had a stroke?

■ 4

The First Visit to the Doctor

If you've been diagnosed with diabetes, your doctor will ask you many questions about your medical history. Because of the time it takes to find out all these important details, this exam may take more than one visit. It will help to write down answers to the questions you'll find in this chapter before you go. Be sure to write down any questions you want to ask the doctor, too.

This medical history will be the foundation for your diabetes care. First, your doctor needs to know when your diabetes first appeared. For those with type I diabetes, this is easier because the symptoms usually occur very dramatically, especially in children and teenagers. For type II diabetes, however, it is more complicated. You may have had it for years, even as long as 10 years, before being diagnosed. This is important because the longer you have had diabetes, the greater your risk for complications.

What Your Doctor Will Ask You

Blood glucose control

There are several ways to figure out blood glucose control from your history. Your doctor will probably ask you questions to find out if you might have the typical symptoms of high blood glucose, called hyperglycemia. These include

- frequent urination (including needing to wake up to go to the bathroom at night)
- frequent thirst
- blurry vision
- weight loss
- vaginal yeast infections

The doctor will also ask about symptoms of hypoglycemia, or low blood glucose. It can be caused by too much insulin, too much sulfonylurea (a pill used to stimulate insulin production), not enough food, or too much exercise. If you have noticed any symptoms that always occur but are not on the following list, tell the doctor:

- hunger
- nervousness
- profuse sweating
- tremor
- seizures or coma

Your doctor will ask you when the symptoms first appeared, how often they appear, and whether you have ever had a blood glucose level so low that you needed assistance from another person. This is called severe hypoglycemia. Someone with a history of hypoglycemia unawareness—having no symptoms when blood glucose levels are dangerously low—will probably have different blood glucose goals from someone without this problem.

Other questions should include:

- Do other family members know what to do if you have an episode of severe hypoglycemia?
- Have they been taught how to use glucagon? (Glucagon is a hormone that causes an increase in blood glucose, and it can be given by injection to treat hypoglycemia.)
- Do you have a glucagon emergency kit readily available?
- Have you checked the date on the container of glucagon to be sure it is not past its expired date?

The doctor will ask about any diabetes-related medications and the doses you are taking.

Self-monitoring of blood glucose

A very important part of your history is SMBG. SMBG gives you information to make your diabetes therapy work better. Many people are never taught how to use blood glucose meters correctly, and everybody should review their technique from time to time. Your doctor may refer you to an ADA-recognized education program or a diabetes educator for this. This person can be a nurse, dietitian, pharmacist, or physician who teaches diabetes self-management skills. Other questions the doctor will ask:

- How frequently do you monitor your blood glucose, and how do you use that information?
- Do you use the glucose results at each reading to adjust your insulin dose or food intake?

- Do you use the glucose results at each reading to change your exercise routine?
- Do you use them to identify specific patterns (such as frequent before-lunch low blood glucose or after-supper high blood glucose)?
- Do you measure blood glucose levels more often for the doctor just before the office visit (or perhaps between visits) to help guide decisions about your diabetes therapy?
- What is your goal for blood glucose levels at different times of the day?

Glycated hemoglobin levels

Glycated hemoglobin tells you about your blood glucose control for the past 12 weeks. The higher the number, the higher the blood glucose levels have been. If possible, bring in the results of your glycated hemoglobin tests for the past several years and the normal ranges for the laboratory that was used. (It's a good idea to keep results of all your tests in your personal records.)

Food

Your doctor will ask about your meal plan and any nutrition education you may have had. Your doctor should ask whether you are eating the same amounts of food at the same meals each day and about the timing of your meals. For instance, are you able to eat only at certain times because of restrictions at work or school? Problems like this should be identified at this first visit. Your doctor may ask what types of food you like and don't like, foods that you seldom eat, and how often you eat foods high in fat or use alcohol. You'll be asked whether you follow a meal plan, count the grams of carbohydrate you eat, or use an exchange system to make food choices. If you've just been diagnosed, your doctor may explain these methods to you and help you select a meal plan or refer you to a nurse educator or dietitian for help. You must have help to set up a meal plan that is fitted to your schedule, the foods you prefer, and your diabetes goals.

Exercise

Exercise is a big part of your diabetes therapy. Your doctor will ask how often and how long you exercise, and how intensely you go at it. Exercise may mean planned physical activity, such as jogging or playing tennis, or it may be exercise you get on the job, such as walking or lifting. You should discuss with your doctor the right shoes and why it's important to inspect your feet after exercise (see Chapters 10 and 11). You'll need to learn how to prevent low blood glucose during and after exercise.

Complications

Some people will spend most of the time during the initial visit discussing complications, both chronic (long lasting) and acute (occurring suddenly). Acute complications include severe hypoglycemia and ketoacidosis (dangerously large quantities of acids called ketones in the urine). Infections are another possible complication, and your doctor should ask about any infections you may have had, including infections of the skin, feet, teeth and gums, and genitals or urinary system (such as kidney, bladder, or vagina).

Eyes

This part of the history should include the following questions:

- When did you last have a dilated eye exam?

- Have you been diagnosed with diabetic retinopathy or visual impairment? If so, when?
- Have you had laser therapy or eye surgery? Chapter 7 covers eye disease in detail.

Kidneys

High blood pressure is linked to diabetic kidney disease (nephropathy). That's why your doctor should know whether you now have or have had high blood pressure and what blood pressure medications you've taken. Your doctor may also ask whether other family members have had high blood pressure or kidney disease, with or without diabetes. If you have records of previous testing for protein in your urine (called albuminuria or proteinuria), bring them along or ask your previous doctor or lab to send the information in advance. Diabetic nephropathy is covered in detail in Chapter 8.

Neuropathy (nerve damage)

Perhaps the most common reason a person with diabetes seeks medical attention is painful neuropathy. You should describe the type of pain (tingling, pins and needles, or cramping) and mention whether you have felt numbness on the bottom of your feet. If you have had foot ulcers, tell the doctor. Supply a list of any medications you used for pain. The doctor should also ask about symptoms that might suggest another type of nerve damage called autonomic neuropathy. Questions might include:

- Do you sometimes feel your heart racing?
- Do you have abdominal bloating and nausea after eating a small amount of food?
- Do you suffer constipation, often alternating with diarrhea?

- Do you become dizzy when you stand up?
- Are you unable to empty your bladder when urinating?
- Do you have sexual dysfunction, such as difficulties maintaining an erection or achieving orgasm?
- Do you sweat after a meal?

For more detail on neuropathy, see Chapter 11.

Circulation problems

Some people with diabetes may have peripheral vascular disease—*plaque* causes a narrowing of the arteries leading to the legs. When not enough blood and oxygen can get to the muscles, you feel pain. The most common symptom is pain or cramping in your calves that develops after activity, such as walking or climbing stairs. Usually the pain goes away after you rest for a few minutes. The medical term for this is *claudication*. Claudication can be measured by how far you walk before the pain develops. For example, for 3 years, you've had pain in your left calf after walking up two flights of stairs, but the pain goes away after a few minutes. That's stable claudication and may not need treatment. If, however, the pain now begins in the left calf after one flight of stairs, this would be progressive claudication. You may need to see a vascular surgeon.

Heart problems

People with diabetes are at high risk for heart problems, so you and your doctor must keep a watchful eye for cardiovascular disease. Things your doctor will need to know:

- Whether you have had a heart attack, bypass surgery, or coronary angioplasty.

- Results of your last electrocardiogram (ECG), stress test, or coronary angiogram.
- Whether you take any medications for heart disease, including aspirin.

Other questions your doctor may ask:
- Do you have chest pain or discomfort, especially with exercise?
- Do you get shortness of breath, perhaps accompanied by sweating?
- Do you have heart palpitations (skipping of heartbeats)?

Many people with diabetes do not have any of these symptoms, however, so checking for risk factors for cardiovascular disease is important. Perhaps the greatest risk is smoking, no matter what type of diabetes you have. One study showed that 68 percent of deaths from heart attack or stroke in men with diabetes could have been prevented if the men had quit smoking and decreased their cholesterol and blood pressure levels.

High levels of two kinds of blood fats, cholesterol and triglycerides, are another known risk factor (see Chapter 10). Ideally you should bring, or have sent to the doctor's office, any tests that measured blood fat (also called lipids). Your doctor will also want to know about any lipid-lowering drugs you may have taken.

Other risk factors your doctor will ask about include how much alcohol you drink, family history of high lipid levels, and family history of premature heart attack (younger than age 60 for men and 70 for women). The other major risk factors are high blood pressure and obesity.

Questions your doctor should ask:
- Do you smoke?
- What are the results of previous lipid (blood fat) tests?
- Have you taken any medication to lower your triglycerides or cholesterol?
- Do other members of your family have high cholesterol or triglycerides?
- Has any male in your family had a heart attack before age 60? Any female before age 70?

Thyroid symptoms

People with type I diabetes have a much higher risk of thyroid disease than the general population, so your doctor may ask you the following questions about symptoms of thyroid problems.

For low thyroid hormone levels (hypothyroidism):
- Are you intolerant to cold?
- Do you have dry skin?
- Is your energy level low?
- (For women) Are your menstrual periods heavy?
- Are you frequently constipated?

For high thyroid hormone levels (hyperthyroidism):
- Are you intolerant to heat?
- Is your heart rate fast?
- Do you get short of breath when you exercise?
- Do you suffer from anxiety or tremors?
- (For women) Are your menstrual periods light or infrequent?
- Do you have loose stools?

Pregnancy

Women newly diagnosed with diabetes may have had diabetes during pregnancy (gestational diabetes) if their babies weighed more than 9 pounds at birth. Any woman with diabetes who is considering getting pregnant should work on excellent blood glucose control with her doctor *before* she gets pregnant. Poorly controlled diabetes can result in serious complications for both the baby and the mother. Because of this, the doctor may also discuss birth control options. (See Chapter 6.)

Cultural issues

Your doctor may ask about cultural issues that can affect your diabetes management. For example, a Mexican American may have different eating or cooking habits from a Japanese American, and these should be included in their diabetes management plan.

Financial considerations

With the cost of daily testing and medications, even routine diabetes care can be expensive. Discuss with your doctor any financial problems that you anticipate. Your doctor should make sure that the cost does not keep you from getting the care you need. For instance, your doctor may reduce your number of daily blood glucose tests by changing the times when you do them, or change your medication to a generic drug. Never alter your treatment on your own because of financial problems. Explain your problem to the doctor so he or she can help you find a safe solution. (See Chapter 12.)

These issues need to be discussed during the first few visits with your doctor.

The Physical Exam

The physical examination should focus on areas where problems usually arise—the eyes, feet, heart, and vascular system. Children with poorly controlled diabetes may not be growing and maturing as they should.

Height and weight
In the initial examination, the doctor will check your weight, and height for children and adolescents. (Weight and height for children will be compared to a growth chart.) Weight changes are an important clue, because they may indicate a change in blood glucose control. A weight gain may suggest a decrease in blood glucose levels. A weight loss suggests poor control with very high blood glucose levels. On the other hand, weight loss also could indicate depression, hyperthyroidism, gastroparesis (a condition in which food doesn't move normally from the stomach into the intestine), and other possibilities.

Blood pressure
High blood pressure, or hypertension, is more common in people with type II diabetes than in the general population and may suggest kidney problems (see Chapter 8). Blood pressure of children and teenagers should be compared to normal blood pressure for their ages. Blood pressure should be measured a bit differently in people with autonomic neuropathy or orthostatic hypotension (a dramatic decrease in blood pressure on standing, accompanied by lightheadedness or even passing out). These people should have their blood pressure and pulse measured first while lying flat and then after standing for 3–5 minutes.

Your doctor can prescribe medication for symptoms related to a large fall in blood pressure.

Eyes

Another important part of the evaluation is examination of the retina. An eye doctor, either an optometrist or ophthalmologist, should also do this. Be sure your eye doctor is aware of your diabetes. (See Chapter 7.)

Internal organs

ADA recommends thyroid examination, heart examination, and abdominal examination (to check for an enlarged liver, which is common in people with type II diabetes).

Pulse

Examination of pulses—the movement of blood thorough an artery—is particularly important. If the doctor cannot feel the pulses in the feet, this strongly suggests a decrease in blood flow and possible vascular disease. Some arteries, if narrowed by plaque, may have an associated sound that can be heard with a stethoscope. This sound is called a "bruit"—from the French word for *noise*. It often occurs in the carotid arteries in the neck and the femoral arteries in the groin. The carotid arteries supply the brain with blood, and the femoral arteries supply the legs.

Feet

Finding and treating foot problems early may prevent complications such as skin ulcers that can lead to infection or even amputation. The doctor should inspect the feet for skin breakdown, calluses, and athlete's foot. All these may lead to infection and ulcers. Areas of redness suggest that shoes fit poorly, and you should be referred to a podiatrist or pedorthist. A pedorthist specializes in fitting shoes properly, particularly for people with a high risk of foot ulcers. A podiatrist specializes in diseases of the feet. (See Chapter 11.)

The doctor should check you for neuropathy (nerve damage). A tuning fork placed on the big toe is an excellent way to check for early neuropathy, because people with neuropathy will feel the vibration stop before it actually does. The absence of an ankle jerk when a reflex hammer is used can also be a sign of diabetic neuropathy, but not for many elderly people. Nylon monofilaments are a popular way to check the foot's ability to feel fine sensation, such as friction from a poor-fitting shoe or a small pebble in your shoe. The doctor will ask you to close your eyes and then ask which toe or part of the foot is being touched with the monofilament. Someone who cannot feel the largest filament on the soles of the feet is at high risk of developing a foot ulcer.

The feet should also be checked for swelling (edema), which may be a sign of kidney or heart disease. Foot deformities such as hammertoes are also common and may increase the risk of skin ulcers. People with neuropathy and foot deformities may be referred to a podiatrist or pedorthist. Fungus in the nails (onychomycosis) is common, and prescription medication is available.

Lab tests
At the first visit, the following laboratory tests are necessary, especially if you haven't had any of them recently:
- Glycated hemoglobin
- Fasting lipid profile, if one has not been done in the last 5 years

- Urine test for microalbuminuria in youngsters past puberty who have had type I diabetes for 5 years, and in everyone with type II diabetes
- Thyroid function studies in anyone with an enlarged thyroid or symptoms of high or low thyroid levels, and everyone with type I diabetes
- ECG (for adults only)

Other tests may be required in certain situations. See Chapters 5 and 10 for more discussion on lipids and Chapters 3 and 8 for more on microalbuminuria.

Building Your Management Plan

Once your doctor has completed your history, the physical exam, and has all your test results, you two can draw up a management plan developed specifically for you. You will manage your diabetes as much as possible—instead of having the doctor do it. You should be closely involved in forming this plan and solving any problems that arise. These problems could include hypoglycemia, irregular mealtimes, or the use of alcohol.

A plan just for you

This plan must take into account your age, school or work schedule, physical activity, eating patterns, social situation and personality, cultural factors, and any diabetes-related complications or other medical conditions you may have. You need to understand each part of the management plan and agree with all care providers about how to follow it. Your goals and plan must fit you and your needs.

Spreading the word

All your other doctors must be notified of your diabetes and treatment plan. Your primary care physician should act as the "quarterback," relaying information to the other doctors and coordinating your care. Sometimes this is complicated; sometimes not. A 28-year-old man with type I diabetes and no complications may only have one other doctor, the ophthalmologist he sees for annual eye exams. His ophthalmologist only needs to know what medications he takes and to check for retinopathy. A 31-year-old pregnant woman with type I diabetes and advanced kidney disease and chest pain, however, may have an obstetrician, a cardiologist, an ophthalmologist, and a nephrologist. All of them will need to know about her treatment plan.

Setting your goals

You need specific short-term and long-term goals. These may include target levels for glycated hemoglobin and SMBG, daily physical activity, stopping smoking, or losing weight. The plan should also be specific about your medications. You need to see a registered dietitian who is familiar with diabetes for help setting up a meal plan. You may also go to a nurse educator to learn how to monitor your blood glucose levels and how to test your urine for ketones.

Eye and foot care

ADA recommends yearly dilated eye exams by an ophthalmologist or optometrist for everyone age 12 and older who have had diabetes for 5 years, all people over the age of 30, and any patient with vision problems (see Chapter 7). Many people will also need to see a podiatrist.

When to call for help

Finally, you should know when and how to contact the doctor or health care team between visits. Your doctor can explain which health problems need to be dealt with immediately and by whom. For instance, mild low blood glucose may not need to be reported to your doctor until the next regular visit. A serious episode with loss of consciousness, however, is an emergency, and 911 or another emergency line should be called right away. You and your doctor must decide when you should come for follow-up and return appointments. Many doctors ask their patients to call, mail, fax, or even e-mail in their blood glucose levels for review between appointments.

The initial encounter with the doctor could sometimes run into several visits. It takes a long time to gather all the necessary information. Be patient! The doctor needs all this information to give you the best possible treatment.

ADA recommendations for continuing care are covered in the rest of this book.

■ 5

Continuing Care

Good continuing care is an essential part of diabetes man
agement. This means regularly scheduled doctor's visits
and sometimes additional contact. For example, if you
have recently started self-monitoring your blood glucose
levels, or had a change in treatment, or if it's so far to the
doctor's office that you have problems getting there, your
doctor may want to talk to you by phone, fax, or e-mail
between office visits.

This may include reporting the results of your home blood
glucose tests, so your doctor can help you make adjustments
in your medication. You can mail this data to your doctor
or fax or e-mail it to save time. (Giving this information
over the phone takes too much time, and it's easy to make
mistakes in copying down the information.)

On the other hand, many doctors do not encourage this
between-visit contact, because they prefer to see you face
to face. Diabetes is so complex, however, that some type

of contact—especially after a major change in treatment plan—is often needed, but an office visit may not be necessary. ADA notes in its Standards of Care that in some situations, such as when a person first starts to inject insulin, daily contact may be needed until the patient's glucose control improves. With a change in diet or oral medication, weekly contact is usually enough.

How Often to Visit

If you are treated with insulin, ADA suggests at least four visits a year to your health care provider. If you do not use insulin, two to four visits are recommended, depending on how you are doing with your treatment goals. More frequent contact may be needed if you aren't meeting your blood glucose or blood pressure goals or if you have symptoms of diabetes-related complications.

Your doctor or nurse educator should have taught you how to recognize problems with your glucose control, based on your blood glucose checks. If you have any concerns with the results of your SMBG, contact your doctor or one of your health care team members. You need a prearranged plan for those problems that require a call to the health care team. For example, ketones in the urine, blood glucose levels persistently above 250 mg/dl, or a blood pressure above 160/100 mmHg all may require contact with the doctor or one of the health care team members.

Reviewing Your Program

Review blood glucose control
At each visit to the doctor, you will repeat some of the

things you did at the first appointment. This includes discussing any hypoglycemia you've had, including frequency, cause, and severity. You should also discuss in detail your blood glucose test results and look for patterns of highs and lows.

Consider computerizing

Many companies that manufacture meters for SMBG have developed computer software to identify patterns in blood glucose levels. For example, a computer program may find a pattern of high before-breakfast blood glucose levels. Some people like pie charts that tell them how many blood glucose levels at a particular time each day are within the target, above the target, or below the target. This type of software will probably become more popular with time, and data from the meters may be downloaded either in the doctor's office or by the patient at home.

Write it down

When reviewing SMBG results, try to find out why a particular blood glucose level was out of range. One of the greatest benefits of SMBG comes from being able to see the effect of a particular type of food, exercise at a specific time of day, a change of medication, or stress. It's best to write this information down, either in a glucose log book or on a piece of paper (most computer software now available cannot record all these data, so it's up to you).

Changes in treatment

At each visit, you should discuss any changes to make in your diabetes care plan. Most often, these are planned changes in medication (especially insulin) for a change in activity, a special celebration dinner, or an abnormal blood glucose result. If you made any change in your treatment plan since your last visit, you should discuss it now.

It is difficult to stick to a treatment plan, for a variety of reasons. Depression, tension at work, or problems at home can all affect your treatment, so it's important to mention them to your doctor. He or she may be able to refer you to outside help, such as a dietitian or a counselor. Financial problems can make it difficult to buy medication and necessary supplies, and your doctor may be able to change your prescription to a less expensive, generic medication or refer you to a social worker to get financial assistance.

Medication and supplies vary greatly in price, so your doctor may advise you to shop around.

Discuss any symptoms

Discuss any symptoms that suggest you are developing complications of diabetes. These could include

- a change in vision—possible retinopathy or cataracts
- swelling of the ankles or painful feet—possible nephropathy
- chest pain—possible heart disease

You should tell your doctor if you have seen another doctor or health care specialist about any problems, if you took any medication, and the name of the medication.

Other health concerns

If you have health problems other than diabetes, you and your doctor should talk about them, too. You may have one doctor who takes care both of your diabetes and other health problems, or you may see one doctor—such as a family doctor or internist—for most of your health care, but go to an endocrinologist for your diabetes.

If you have more than one doctor, it's important that everyone is clear about which doctor does what. For instance, you may have one doctor who manages your diabetes, another who prescribes medication for high blood pressure, and a third who is responsible for routine immunizations. This is critical, because all too often, more than one doctor is prescribing different medications for the same problem. Or one doctor may prescribe a medicine that should not be taken with one prescribed by a second doctor. One drug could interfere with the effects of another or cause a dangerous interaction. Even if your doctor doesn't ask, always tell him or her about any medications you are taking. Some people find it helpful to bring all the bottles of medications that they are taking to the appointment with them.

All your health care providers must talk to each other to ensure that you're getting the best possible care. In many large clinics, university hospitals, or certain health maintenance organizations (HMOs), this may be less of a problem, because one medical chart is used by all of the providers.

Physical Exam

ADA recommends that parts of the physical exam be repeated at all your visits. At every visit, weight and blood pressure should be measured, and height of children. Anything that was abnormal on previous visits needs to be checked. For instance, on the previous visit, your doctor may have found a large callus on the bottom of your foot and told you to use a pumice stone to try to decrease its size or may have treated a skin infection with antibiotics. Now your doctor will want to check the callus and make sure that the infection has cleared up.

Feet

Your feet should be examined at every visit. If the foot exam reveals poor circulation, loss of sensation, deformity, ulceration, or infection, your doctor may refer you to a specialist such as a podiatrist. The doctor or a nurse educator may explain clearly how to inspect your feet and how to take care of them. Your doctor may also give you pamphlets about foot care.

Eyes

Your doctor should check your retinas for retinopathy. ADA recommends that a dilated eye exam be done annually by an ophthalmologist or optometrist for

- all people age 10 and older who have had diabetes for 5 years
- everyone over the age of 30
- any patient with visual symptoms and/or abnormalities

The eye doctor will check your eyes for cataracts and glaucoma as well as retinopathy. Vision loss from diabetes may result from any of these three eye diseases. The annual eye exams are crucial, because many eye problems, if caught early, can be treated. Of all the blind people in the United States, 8 percent became blind because of diabetes, and approximately 12 percent of new cases of blindness are due to diabetes. Screening and early treatment can help save your sight. (See Chapter 7.)

Ongoing Lab Work

The following lab tests are needed regularly.

Glycated hemoglobin

This test measures blood glucose control for the previous 12–16 weeks. People treated with insulin should have this test quarterly. People who do not use insulin need it two to four times a year or as frequently as needed to check how close you are to your blood glucose goals. The glycated hemoglobin level may help motivate you and improve blood glucose control, because it lets you know your blood glucose levels over a period of weeks. To best use this information, however, you need to hear the results of the test during or shortly after the visit to the doctor. (If you have to wait 3 months until your next visit, you won't be able to make the best use of this important test.) Many doctors use a glycated hemoglobin test that supplies the result in less than 10 minutes. The blood is drawn at the beginning of the visit, and the results are available by the time the doctor discusses your diabetes control with you.

Fasting blood glucose

This test, done at your doctor's office or in the laboratory, measures the glucose in your blood in the morning when you haven't eaten since the previous evening. It helps determine diabetes control in people with type II diabetes, particularly those who do not perform SMBG. For those who do, it's a good idea to check your blood glucose within 5 minutes of the laboratory blood glucose test to check your meter for accuracy. You may find, for example, that your meter gives you results that are higher than the lab results. If this happens every time, you can adjust for this difference when you are doing glucose checks at home.

Lipid (blood fat) levels

Lipid levels deserve special attention from people with diabetes (see Chapter 10). ADA recommends that adults with abnormal lipid test results be tested yearly for the following types of blood fats:

- total cholesterol
- HDL (high-density lipoprotein) cholesterol
- LDL (low-density lipoprotein) cholesterol
- fasting triglycerides

If you have abnormal lipid levels—high triglycerides, high LDL and total cholesterol, or low HDL cholesterol—your doctor will recommend changes in the food you eat and, perhaps, in medication. Your lipid levels should be tested as necessary to see whether your treatment is working. If the lipid measurements fall within normal ranges, you may not need tests so often. For children with type I diabetes, the lipid levels should be measured after age 2. If the levels are abnormal or borderline, the test should be repeated to be sure of the results. Children with normal lipid levels should have another test in 5 years.

Urine albumin

Large amounts of albumin, a type of protein, in the urine may indicate kidney disease (see Chapter 8). People who are past puberty and have had type I diabetes for at least 5 years should have this test. People with type II diabetes should be tested soon after diagnosis, because they may have had diabetes for years before being diagnosed.

Management Plan

At each visit, review your management plan to find problems and check your progress in meeting your goals. For most people with diabetes, this will include a review of
- diabetes control (including exercise)
- complications
- blood pressure control
- lipid levels
- frequency of hypoglycemia

You may need to be referred to specialists, such as an endocrinologist for diabetes control, an ophthalmologist for eye exams, or a nephrologist for advanced kidney disease. Your skills in managing your diabetes should be looked at once a year. You and your health care provider need to review any medication you take, food and exercise changes you can make based on your daily blood glucose checks, routine foot care, meal planning, treatment of hypoglycemia, and any other element of successful diabetes care.

It may not be possible for every doctor to provide care that meets the ADA Standards of Care. Reasons range from patient insurance that does not cover SMBG, or the lack of a diabetes educator to instruct patients, to a doctor not being experienced in all the facets of treating a person with diabetes. In these instances, ADA suggests you be referred to one of the following:

- an endocrinologist (a doctor who specializes in diseases of the endocrine system, which includes the pancreas, which secretes insulin)
- a treatment team led by a diabetologist (an endocrinologist who specializes in treating diabetes)

Questions to Ask Your Doctor

Should I send in my SMBG results?

What SMBG results should trigger an immediate call to you or a member of my health care team? Whom should I call?

Where can I get a computer program to identify blood glucose levels from my SMBG? What should I look for in such a program?

Who should I call when I have a question? What if it is on a weekend?

Is there anything new in diabetes treatment?

What should I do if I want to greatly increase my exercise?

How can I adhere to my meal plan when I eat out? When I'm at a party?

Do I need to see an eye doctor? Who should I see?

Questions Your Doctor May Ask You

Have you had any change in your vision? chest pain? ankle swelling? painful feet?

Have you seen another doctor?

Are you taking any other medication?

Have you seen an optometrist or ophthalmologist?

Have you increased (or decreased) the amount you exercise?

Have you had problems sticking to your treatment plan?

Have you had any problems with hypoglycemia?

You may not be able to get a referral to a specialist. Specialists are not available in all communities. Also, a primary care provider may not understand your need to be referred. In a managed-care insurance plan, you may be responsible for paying the diabetologist. These concerns are discussed in Chapter 12.

■ 6

Pregnancy

Pregnant women with diabetes are classified into two categories: those who had diabetes before pregnancy and those whose diabetes develops during the pregnancy, which is called gestational diabetes. Gestational diabetes goes away after the baby is born.

Because of possible harm to the baby, women with diabetes who plan to become pregnant must work with their doctor and diabetes team to keep their diabetes under careful control. With insulin for those who need it and the tools for good blood glucose control, we can lower the risks to both mother and baby. Careful control before and during pregnancy is crucial.

For Preexisting Diabetes

Both type I and type II diabetes can affect the baby's development in the womb. In African American women over age 30, type II diabetes complicates pregnancy more often than type I diabetes. In general, the better the diabetes control of the mother, the fewer complications in the baby. Poor diabetes control appears to cause birth defects in the developing baby in the first few weeks after conception. Later in the pregnancy, high blood glucose levels result in other complications: large babies, babies whose lungs do not work properly after birth, and babies with hypoglycemia after delivery. These problems can result in a difficult birth, longer hospital stays for the baby, or, in worst cases, death of the baby.

What can go wrong

Miscarriages occur more often in women with preexisting diabetes. Another major concern is birth defects, which occur as the baby develops in the womb. The way to handle these scary statistics is to get your diabetes under excellent control before you become pregnant. Careful blood glucose control before pregnancy can dramatically decrease the risk of birth defects. The risk of these problems occurring in a woman with excellent blood glucose control is less than 5 percent, close to the risk in a woman who does not have diabetes. This means that, with careful diabetes care, the risk to your baby will be little more than the risk of any pregnant woman.

Your baby's major organs—heart, brain, kidneys—are already formed 6 weeks into your pregnancy (the 8th week after your last menstrual period). Poorly controlled diabetes in the early weeks of pregnancy, often before a woman even knows that she is pregnant, greatly increases the risk of either a miscarriage or a baby with a major malformation. There is a connection between glycated hemoglobin level and the risk of miscarriage and birth defects: the higher the mother's glycated hemoglobin, the higher the risk to the baby's health.

Counseling should begin early

Because of the possible risks for both mother and child, some doctors begin prepregnancy counseling around the time of a young woman's first menstrual period, when she is 11 or 12 years old. Women in their child-bearing years, and teenagers in particular, should regularly discuss contraceptive needs and any concerns about future pregnancy with their health care team.

Medications you can't take

There are medications you cannot use during pregnancy. These include all the oral medications for diabetes, including sulfonylureas, metformin (Glucophage), and acarbose (Precose). You will need to stop using these drugs *before* you get pregnant. You must consult with your doctor about this. Your doctor may switch you to insulin for the time that you are pregnant. (See Appendix 1.) Antidepressants or other medications may also need to be discontinued during the pregnancy, so you should tell your doctor about every medication you're taking, including over-the-counter drugs.

Measuring the risks

To determine the risks to both you and the developing baby, you will need some tests. You'll be examined by an ophthalmologist or optometrist (because retinopathy may worsen during pregnancy), have microalbuminuria and kidney function checked (see Chapter 8), and have an electrocardiogram (ECG). Your glycated hemoglobin should be tested regularly, and you will need to learn SMBG for testing at home. Some pregnant women may test as often as 8 times a day to maintain good control.

Reviewing the treatment plan

Blood glucose control is crucial for a healthy pregnancy for mother and child. If you have type I diabetes and are considering pregnancy, you need to understand all of the principles of intensive diabetes management—nutrition counseling, frequent SMBG, regular exercise, and how to adjust insulin doses as needed. You will need to see a dietitian and also get advice about your exercise program before you become pregnant.

Stress

Pregnancy may cause tremendous emotional stress for some women. Your relationship with your partner can relieve the stress or make it worse, and the doctor may ask questions about this. In some situations, you may see a mental health professional, especially if you have a history of depression and your antidepressants are discontinued during the pregnancy. Financial stresses must also be considered. Pregnancy for a woman with type I diabetes can be quite expensive, and it's best to deal with questions about insurance coverage before you get pregnant.

Life expectancy and complications

One of the most common questions women with diabetes ask is how pregnancy affects their life expectancy. The answer for women with type I diabetes is there appears to be no effect, except for those with known coronary artery disease (see Chapters 4 and 10). Pregnancy is not usually life threatening. However, women with diabetes do have a greater risk for the following complications:

- Ketoacidosis—a life-threatening emergency. The body burns fats when it can't get enough glucose (you're not eating enough or not taking enough insulin). Ketones, a waste product of the breakdown of fats, are acids that can be extremely dangerous in large quantities.
- Preeclampsia—high blood pressure caused by pregnancy, which can pose risks to both mother and developing baby.
- Cesarean sections—partly because diabetic women tend to have large babies.

Eye problems

Stable proliferative retinopathy that has been treated with laser therapy and nonproliferative retinopathy do not usually get worse during pregnancy. If you don't have diabetic retinopathy, you probably will not develop it during pregnancy. On the other hand, active proliferative retinopathy that has not been treated with laser therapy may get much worse during pregnancy. That's why it's best to wait until the retinopathy has been treated and is stable before trying to get pregnant.

Kidney disease (nephropathy)

The effect pregnancy has on nephropathy depends on how damaged the kidneys are. Women with protein in their urine, but normal kidney function, may find that their kidneys get worse during pregnancy—they will return to normal after the baby is born. More advanced kidney disease can be harmful to the mother and baby, causing complications such as early delivery and a smaller-than-normal baby. Signs that these complications might occur are

- more than 3 grams of protein in the urine per day in the first trimester or more than 10 grams per day in the third trimester
- a serum creatinine (measure of kidney function) level greater than 1.5 mg/dl at the start of pregnancy
- high blood pressure
- severe anemia

Home testing is essential

Blood glucose goals. Your blood glucose goals during pregnancy should be as close to a nondiabetic woman's glucose levels as possible. This is often difficult because insulin requirements keep changing during pregnancy. For example, toward the end of the first trimester, insulin requirements commonly go down by 10–20 percent. But, after 18–24 weeks of pregnancy, insulin requirements usually increase. In addition, blood glucose control is difficult with morning sickness. You may take your insulin, but if the food doesn't stay in your stomach, and this creates a risk for hypoglycemia. Vomiting can also cause ketosis—the accumulation of the acids known as ketones—which can be dangerous and must be avoided during pregnancy. That is why pregnant women with preexisting diabetes often need to monitor their blood glucose levels 8 times a day to reach their targets (see Table 6–1). You want your glycated hemoglobin to be in the upper range of normal. For example, if the normal range for glycated hemoglobin is 4.0–6.0 percent, the goal for a diabetic pregnancy would be 6.0 percent. The glycated hemoglobin level should be measured every 4–6 weeks to check on your diabetes control.

Ketones in the urine. The other important test that needs to be done at home is testing for urine ketones. If you don't

Table 6–1
Blood Glucose Goals in Diabetic Pregnancy

Fasting	60–90 mg/dl
Premeal	60–105 mg/dl
1 hour postmeal	110–130 mg/dl
2 hours postmeal	90–120 mg/dl
2–6 AM	60–120 mg/dl

eat enough calories for your and the growing baby's needs, you may find ketones in your urine, which is a sign of starvation. Ketones in the urine are also in the blood and may be dangerous to the developing nervous system of the baby. You may need to make changes in diet or insulin or both. Ketones are most likely to be present when you first wake up, because this is the longest period you go without food. This is an important time to test. Your doctor will tell you what levels to watch for. Urine ketone testing is also important if you miss a meal or eat later than usual, with any illness, or with any blood glucose test above 200 mg/dl. Ketones in the urine (called ketonuria) may be the first sign of an infection preceding ketoacidosis. Ketoacidosis usually develops gradually, so be on the lookout for symptoms of it. Mothers with ketoacidosis have a 50–90 percent chance of losing the baby.

ADA published guidelines in 1996 for how often women with preexisting diabetes should have certain tests during pregnancy (Table 6–2). Routine thyroid function testing is also recommended for women with type I diabetes because it is so common for them.

Table 6–2
Frequency of Testing During Pregnancy for Women With Preexisting Diabetes

Test	Frequency
Glycated hemoglobin	Every 4–6 weeks
Glucose	Fingerstick at home, 4–8 times daily
Fasting ketone	Daily
Kidney function: 24-hour urine for total protein and creatinine clearance	Each trimester
Eye status	1st trimester and then as necessary
Thyroid function	Baseline; repeat as needed

Gestational Diabetes

Diabetes that develops during pregnancy is called gestational diabetes. Two to 3 percent of pregnant women are diagnosed with gestational diabetes.

When to test

ADA recommends that all pregnant women be screened for gestational diabetes at 24–28 weeks after conception. This does not need to be a fasting test. If your blood glucose 1 hour after drinking the 50-gram glucose drink is above 140 mg/dl, you will be asked to take a 100-gram 3-hour oral glucose tolerance test (Table 6–3). The 3-hour test is done after an overnight fast of 8–14 hours and after 3 days of carbohydrate loading. The test is designed for these conditions and, if it is not done this way, it will give inaccurate results. During these tests, your blood glucose must be measured by a lab, not by a fingerstick glucose measurement with a meter. The lab checks plasma glucose, while the fingerstick test you do at home checks blood in the small blood vessels called capillaries.

What can go wrong
Fortunately, if gestational diabetes is diagnosed and managed, nothing much goes wrong. However, without proper care during pregnancy, women with gestational diabetes may have some problems. The two most common complications are large babies and hypoglycemia in the baby immediately after birth. The baby will need to be given glucose in a vein. These complications occur because glucose from the mother freely crosses the placenta and causes the developing baby to secrete extra insulin. With extra glucose and insulin, the baby gains more weight than usual. The baby's extra insulin causes hypoglycemia after birth because the glucose from the mother has been turned off.

Table 6–3
Criteria for Diagnosis of Gestational Diabetes

	Time of Testing			
	Fasting	1 hour	2 hour	3 hour
Plasma Glucose	105 mg/dl	190 mg/dl	165 mg/dl	145 mg/dl

Gestational diabetes is diagnosed if 2 or more of these plasma glucose levels are met or exceeded.

Goal 1: normal blood glucose

If you have gestational diabetes, your first goal is to achieve normal blood glucose levels. These may be defined as

- fasting plasma glucose below 105 mg/dl
- 1 hour aftermeal plasma glucose below 140 mg/dl (this test is done in the lab)
- 2 hours aftermeal blood glucose below 120 mg/dl

Goal 2: eating well

The second goal is to eat enough good foods. Your food choices should include all of the essential nutrients the baby needs plus all you need to maintain good health. You want the weight you gain to be healthy weight, and you want to avoid ketonuria.

Your doctor may consider putting you on insulin if your meal plan does not bring your fasting blood glucose below 90 mg/dl or 1 hour aftermeal blood glucose below 120 mg/dl most of the time. If you are starting insulin for the first time, a qualified diabetes educator should teach you how. You'll need to know the basic timing and action of insulin, how to give yourself injections, adjustments to make to your meal plan, and how to recognize and treat hypoglycemia.

Will it reoccur?

If you have had gestational diabetes once, you have a 65 percent chance of developing it in future pregnancies. Also, your chance of developing type II diabetes in the next 5–15 years ranges from 40 to 60 percent. It is recommended that every woman who has had gestational diabetes have a yearly blood glucose measurement. Once you have weaned the baby, you will want to lose the weight you gained with the pregnancy. Returning to a healthy weight

Healthy Eating for a Healthy Infant

Meal planning is the most important part of gestational diabetes therapy. You should develop your own meal plan with a dietitian, but these are recommendations for everyone:

- Avoid sweets. This includes candy, pastries, soft drinks, cookies, and ice cream. They give you few nutrients but a lot of calories.
- Avoid convenience foods, such as hamburgers, fries, and pizza, because they tend to be high in fat.
- Eat 5 or 6 small meals instead of 3 big ones—this keeps aftermeal blood glucose levels down and may help with nausea and heartburn, common complaints during pregnancy.
- Protein foods are absorbed more slowly than carbohydrates like bread, potatoes, starchy vegetables, beans, pasta, and fruit. Good choices include low-fat meats such as turkey, chicken, or lean beef; tofu; low-fat yogurt or cottage cheese; fish; and legumes (dried beans and peas).
- Try eating a small breakfast, because blood glucose levels tend to rise higher after breakfast. Test to see what effect fruit or juice with breakfast has on your blood glucose.
- Choose high-fiber foods such as whole-grain breads, oatmeal, beans, and raw fruits and vegetables. They cause blood glucose to rise more slowly after a meal.
- Limit fatty foods such as pastries, sausage, bacon, butter, salad dressing, and nuts. Per gram, they have twice as many calories as protein or carbohydrate. They make you and the baby gain weight and can cause higher blood glucose levels.

and getting regular exercise will help you prevent getting type II diabetes in the future.

Avoiding Unplanned Pregnancies

Because an unplanned pregnancy could be so devastating to a woman with any type of diabetes, contraception is crucial. There is no best method for all women with diabetes. Each has advantages and drawbacks.

The pill

Oral contraceptives (birth control pills) contain either estrogen plus progestin or progestin only. The combination pill can increase your insulin requirement and raise your blood pressure. Today, oral contraceptives have lower doses of hormones than in the past. However, the estrogen in some pills may increase the risk of a blood clot in a vein, a stroke, or a heart attack, particularly in older women and those who smoke. If you smoke or are older than 35, you should avoid contraceptives that combine estrogen and progestin. High blood pressure is also considered a reason not to use a birth control pill that contains estrogen.

If a combined contraceptive is used, ask about one with a low dose of estrogen (less than or equal to 35 micrograms) and a low dose of progestin. The progestin-only pills do not have a great risk associated with them but are a little less effective. A new combination pill with a progestin called norgestimate and low levels of a synthetic estrogen seems to work best for women with diabetes.

Norplant

The Norplant system is another option. Six small capsules

inserted under the skin of the upper arm release progestin slowly and steadily. The capsules may be effective for 5 years. The major disadvantage is irregular menstrual periods in one in four women. It will change your insulin requirements, and you will need to check with your health care team often to make insulin adjustments.

Depo-Provera

Depo-Provera, a progestin, is injected every 3 months and is highly effective. Irregular bleeding may be troublesome at first, but after 1 year of use, most women cease having menstrual periods. Your insulin requirements will change, and you will need to make insulin adjustments with your health care team.

Diaphragm

The diaphragm, when used correctly with spermicide jelly, carries no medical risks. It is a barrier method of birth control. This method could be 98 percent effective if women use it correctly. This method is frequently chosen by women with diabetes who want to delay childbearing or the time between babies and are not ready for permanent sterilization methods.

Condoms

The condom, used with spermicidal foam, is another barrier method and is about as effective as the diaphragm. Latex condoms also offer protection against a number of sexually transmitted diseases.

Other options

Table 6–4 gives information about birth control options. Intrauterine devices (IUDs) are effective, but one study

Table 6–4
Contraceptive Methods for Diabetic Women

Type	Effectiveness (%)
Oral contraceptive	
Combined estrogen and progestin	98
Progestin only	94
Norplant System	99
Depo-Provera	99
Barrier methods	
Diaphragm + spermicide	98
Condom + foam	88
Intrauterine devices	
Progesterone containing	97
Copper containing	97
Rhythm	80
Sterilization	99+

indicated a higher failure rate in women with diabetes than in women who did not have diabetes. There is also a risk of pain, irregular bleeding, perforation of the uterus, and infection. Because of the risk of infection, IUDs are not usually recommended for women with diabetes. The rhythm method has an effectiveness rate of 75–80 percent—not reliable enough to recommend for women with diabetes.

Permanent methods
If you are sure you will not want any more children, you may choose to have your tubes tied, or your partner may opt for a vasectomy. In particular, women with advanced

complications of diabetes, such as kidney or eye disease or nerve damage, may choose one of these options. With advanced complications, pregnancy is often more difficult. With advanced kidney disease, it is extremely difficult.

■ 7

Diabetic Eye Disease

Your eyesight is precious, and it's true that diabetes can threaten your vision. Diabetes is the leading cause of new cases of blindness in people ages 20–74 in the United States. About 8 percent of Americans who are legally blind have diabetes. Approximately 12 percent of people who have had type I diabetes for 30 years or more are blind. Diabetic eye disease has a tremendous cost—$500 million yearly.

But you are not powerless. You can help protect your vision. Three major eye problems cause people with diabetes to lose their eyesight: diabetic retinopathy, cataracts, and glaucoma. All of them can be avoided or their impact lessened with treatment if they are diagnosed early. Your best weapon against eye disease is an eye doctor with experience in treating these diseases. Visit this eye doctor at least once a year and contact him or her immediately when problems arise or you have any sudden change in vision.

Retinopathy

Your eyes are hollow globes with a diameter of about 1 inch. Light entering the eye is first focused by the cornea and then by the lens (Figure 7–1). This light forms an image on the retina, a multilayered structure lining the back wall of the eye. Light must pass through all the cells of the retina to reach special cells called photoreceptors. The retina also contains the optic disk, or blind spot, which is the junction of nerve fibers that relay information to the brain.

Retinopathy means disease of the retina. As we learned from the DCCT, careful blood glucose control can lower your chances of getting this serious eye disease. In the DCCT, fewer people who followed the intensive regimen had retinopathy. Those who did have retinopathy had milder cases.

Nonproliferative retinopathy

One type of retinopathy is "background," or *nonproliferative* retinopathy. Nonproliferative retinopathy can first be detected with the use of an ophthalmoscope (an instrument with a bright light used to look into the back of the eye). Your doctor will see microaneurisms, tiny red dots, that are actually pouches on the blood vessels. Your eye doctor may also find something called hard exudates, which are yellowish white deposits of protein material that often glisten when viewed through the ophthalmoscope.

While nonproliferative retinopathy can cause blurry vision, it only seriously affects vision if it affects the macula, the center of the retina that gives us sharp vision.

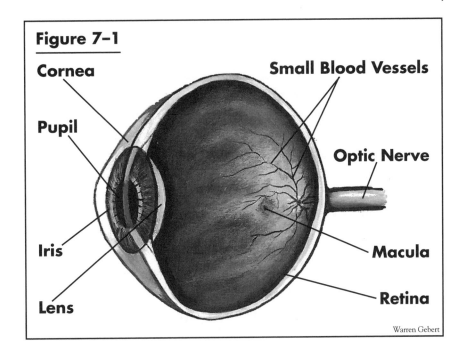

Figure 7-1

Cornea

Pupil

Iris

Lens

Small Blood Vessels

Optic Nerve

Macula

Retina

Warren Gebert

Macular edema is the swelling or thickening of the macula, which is next to the optic nerve head (see Figure 7–1). Vision is particularly affected when the central part of the macula is involved. This condition is difficult to see with the ophthalmoscope and must be diagnosed by an eye doctor with more sophisticated instruments. Each year, about 95,000 Americans with diabetes will develop macular edema, which can limit vision and even lead to blindness. Fortunately, macular edema can be treated with laser surgery (see below).

Proliferative retinopathy

Proliferative retinopathy involves growth of new blood vessels. These new vessels can form near or on the optic disk or elsewhere on the retina. These new vessels are quite fragile and can break, causing significant bleeding. Occasionally, this bleeding can cause the retina to detach from the eye. Proliferative retinopathy, with or without retinal detachment, can damage your vision. Around 84,000 Americans will develop proliferative retinopathy each year. Nearly half of those will develop proliferative retinopathy severe enough to cause vision loss. Fortunately, treatment with laser surgery can dramatically improve the chances of regaining your vision. If the retina has detached or bled a lot, surgery called *vitrectomy* can remove the blood and scar tissue that impairs the vision, and repair the retina.

Advanced diabetic retinopathy poses a significant risk of loss of vision. One large study, the Diabetes Retinopathy Study, showed that advanced proliferative retinopathy resulted in a 25–40 percent risk of severe vision loss over a 2-year period. However, laser therapy decreased this risk by about 60 percent. An ophthalmologist aims a laser (an intense beam of light) at the retina and makes 1,200–1,600 or more tiny burns throughout the retina, except the macula. Laser therapy may cause a minor decrease in vision, but the potential benefits can outweigh the risks.

Cataracts

The second major cause of vision loss is cataracts, a cloudiness of the lens, which is normally clear and transparent. Cataracts are particularly frequent in older people with diabetes. However, cataracts do occur at a younger age and get worse faster if a person has diabetes. In one large study, cataracts caused more decrease in vision than retinopathy in people who developed diabetes after age 30. The greatest risks for the development of cataracts include age, how long you have had diabetes, and how well you control your blood glucose.

Treatment of cataracts in people with diabetes is the same as that used for those without diabetes. Use of sunglasses may relieve visual symptoms. If surgery is required (either with or without lens implantation), it restores vision in 90–95 percent of cases.

Glaucoma

The third major source of vision loss in people with diabetes is *glaucoma*. This is particularly more common with type II diabetes. This vision loss is due to nerve damage from increased pressure in the eye, which is more common in people with diabetes. It occurs in 1–2 percent of people over 60 who do not have diabetes. In people diagnosed with diabetes after age 30, the rate is 7–12 percent. This disease has no symptoms other than the slow loss of the peripheral and central fields of vision. Some people with developing glaucoma compensate for the lack of peripheral vision by turning their heads more to see and are initially not even aware of this vision loss. The most common type of glaucoma, open-angle glaucoma, is effectively treated with eyedrops (for example, pilocarpine, carbachol, and timolol). Occasionally, people need oral medication if the eyedrops do not decrease the pressure enough.

How Often Should Your Eyes Be Checked?

ADA has developed recommendations for the frequency of eye examinations. Have a comprehensive dilated eye and visual examination yearly. If you have retinopathy, you should be referred to an experienced ophthalmologist.

People with type I diabetes

You should be screened each year for retinopathy, beginning 5 years after your diabetes began. Usually, screening doesn't need to be done before the start of puberty, because retinopathy is rare in young people.

People with type II diabetes

You should have an initial examination for retinopathy shortly after the diagnosis of diabetes. If tested by dilated ophthalmoscopy—or if you have persistent high glucose levels of protein in the urine—you should have annual exams by an eye specialist experienced in managing diabetic retinopathy. If tested by a procedure that involves reading 7-field stereophotographs and no retinopathy is found at the first exam, the next test can be repeated in 4 years but should be done yearly after that.

Women with diabetes who become pregnant

You should have a comprehensive eye examination in the first trimester and close follow-up throughout pregnancy. This does not apply to women with gestational diabetes, because they are not at increased risk for retinopathy.

People who already have eye disease

If you have significant macular edema, moderate to severe nonproliferative retinopathy, or proliferative retinopathy, you need immediate care by an ophthalmologist experienced in treating diabetic retinopathy.

These recommendations are based on research that has shown how well treatment works when it is begun before the disease progresses too far. Unfortunately, these recommendations are often not followed. Many studies can be summarized by saying that Americans with diabetes, overall, fall far short of meeting the annual eye exam recommendations.

How to Select an Eye Doctor

You'll want an eye care specialist who knows about diabetes and the eye problems associated with it. Here's a brief guide to eye specialists:

Ophthalmologists—medical doctors who specialize in eye diseases. They can treat eye problems with medicines and can do surgery.

Optometrists—people trained in checking for common eye problems, such as farsightedness or nearsightedness. They are not medical doctors and cannot perform surgery. In some states, they cannot prescribe medications.

Retina specialists—ophthalmologists with special training in diagnosing and treating retina diseases.

ADA recommends you see an ophthalmologist if you have
- unexplained vision problems, such as spots, floaters, blind spots, eye pain
- deterioration in sharpness of vision
- increased intraocular pressure, which another doctor may test for
- any retina abnormality
- retinopathy

In a large 1989 U.S. study, only 69 percent of people with type I diabetes and 61 percent with type II diabetes reported having an eye examination within the past year. In another large study reported in 1994 by investigators at the National Institutes of Health, only 44–57 percent of all people with diabetes had ever had a dilated eye exam. (This exam is recommended yearly for most people with diabetes.) Many other studies have shown even worse results. For example, a 1995 study reported that only 22

Questions to Ask Your Doctor

How often should I have an eye exam?

What symptoms should I look for between exams?

Should I wear sunglasses to help prevent cataracts? What type of sunglasses?

At what age should my eye doctor begin checking for glaucoma?

How do I find an eye doctor experienced in treating diabetic complications?

Are contact lenses harmful?

What is the best eye protection to wear for racquetball? Do I need eye protection for other sports?

Is radial keratomy safe for me?

Does night vision get worse with retinopathy?

How does high or low blood glucose affect my vision?

Questions Your Doctor May Ask You

When was your last eye exam? Did you have your eyes dilated?

Were you tested for glaucoma?

Was retinopathy found?

When did the eye doctor want to see you again?

Were pictures taken of your retina?

percent of diabetic people in a California HMO were referred for eye screening.

The results are quite clear. Diabetes-related eye disease may result in significant loss of vision and blindness. Fortunately, proper screening and treatment can reduce or prevent much of this vision loss. Unfortunately, two things can keep screening and treatment from happening. One is lack of knowledge by both patients and doctors. The other is that eye screening is yet another expense that many people are not willing to take on. Laser surgery can also be quite expensive. On the other hand, severe visual loss that will occur without screening and treatment has high costs, too. One of the major health issues for the next century will be how we can pay for diabetes-related eye disease.

■ 8

Diabetic Nephropathy

Your kidneys work 24 hours a day to clean your blood of toxins that you may take in or that are made in the body. In diabetic kidney disease, called nephropathy, the blood vessels that carry the toxins to the kidneys become blocked and leaky. The result is that some toxins remain in the blood, and some protein that should remain is removed. Unfortunately, kidneys work so well that, by the time you notice problems, as much as 80 percent of your kidneys may be damaged.

When the kidneys completely fail, no medication can help. The only ways to treat kidney failure, also called end stage renal disease, is with dialysis or a kidney transplant. Dialysis is a method of cleaning the blood with an artificial kidney or a machine. Several types are available. Kidney transplants are generally more effective, but a suitable kidney must be available, and you would have to take drugs to keep the body's immune system from rejecting the new kidney. A transplant offers an opportunity for a normal lifestyle, but there are risks and drawbacks.

Obviously, the best thing to do is to focus on keeping your kidneys working. Unfortunately, diabetes now accounts for more than a third of all kidney failure in the United States, and people with diabetes are the fastest-growing group of dialysis and transplant recipients. The cost for this treatment in 1991 was more than $2 billion. A similar upswing in diabetes-linked kidney failure is occurring in other countries. Worldwide, an estimated 100,000 people with diabetes are either receiving dialysis or have had a kidney transplant.

Because of an explosion of research about diabetic nephropathy during the last 10 years, we now better understand the risks of this disease and how to manage it. This has resulted in better early treatment programs, which may prevent or slow the disease. ADA has developed specific standards for the treatment of diabetic nephropathy.

Who's at Risk

Several things contribute to the risk of developing diabetic nephropathy. The longer a person has had diabetes, the higher the risk of kidney disease. But, after 40 years, only 30–50 percent of people with type I diabetes develop diabetic kidney disease. This suggests that how long you have diabetes is not all that influences when or even whether you get nephropathy.

Blood glucose control

One of the most important risk factors is blood glucose control. The better your blood glucose control, the less your chance of developing nephropathy. This has been confirmed in many studies, both in people with type I and those with type II diabetes.

Genetic factors

Genetic factors also may play an important role in development of nephropathy. Nephropathy is more likely to occur in a person with diabetes if a brother or sister has diabetic nephropathy.

High blood pressure

If you have hypertension (high blood pressure), you have a greater risk for nephropathy. In addition, diabetic children of nondiabetic parents with high blood pressure are more likely to have kidney disease.

Smoking and high cholesterol

Other reported risk factors include smoking and high cholesterol levels. It is well known that people with advanced diabetic nephropathy have elevated cholesterol levels.

What Happens to Your Kidneys

Because type I diabetes comes on in a dramatic way, it's pretty clear when it begins. The exact beginning of type II diabetes, however, is usually unknown. Therefore, we have a better understanding of how nephropathy develops in people with type I diabetes.

Early warning tests

Typically, in type I diabetes, soon after the diabetes is diagnosed, the kidney weight and size increase. This goes along with an increase in glomerular filtration rate (GFR), a test that measures kidney function. Normal GFR is about 120 ml/min. A GFR of 150 ml/min shows that a person with type I diabetes may be susceptible to diabetic nephropathy. An improvement in blood glucose control, however, can reduce the GFR to normal.

During the first 2–3 years after the diagnosis of type I diabetes, kidneys often show microscopic evidence of diabetic nephropathy, and GFR stays high. Usually after 10–15 years, small amounts of a type of protein called albumin is lost in the urine. *Microalbuminuria* is the term used when kidneys lose albumin in quantities too small to be detected on the dipstick used in most clinical laboratories. Microalbuminuria is defined as 30–300 mg of albumin in a 24-hour urine collection.

Patients with type I diabetes and microalbuminuria are at a higher risk of developing advanced nephropathy and end-stage renal disease. However, levels of microalbuminuria can vary from day to day, and a variety of things may make albumin levels look high. These include poor diabetes control, infection, exercise, and blood from a menstrual period. Correcting or changing these things will reduce or get rid of the albumin in the urine. So, a doctor will need to know several things about the collected urine before diagnosing a problem with high albumin. Also, because microalbuminuria levels can vary widely from day to day, anyone with abnormal results needs repeat tests.

The next step
If left untreated, albumin levels in the urine will continue to increase, and eventually blood pressure levels will rise as well. Once albumin in the urine exceeds 300 mg per day, the dipstick used to analyze urine in most laboratories will measure it too. This stage is therefore called dipstick-positive proteinuria, or clinical nephropathy. (*Proteinuria*

refers to all proteins, including albumin. Generally, 300 mg of albumin equals about 500 mg of protein in the urine.)

By this stage, the GFR is usually no longer elevated. Without treatment, protein in the urine will continue to increase and GFR to decrease. Blood pressure and cholesterol levels may become extremely high, anemia may develop, and the ankles and hands may become swollen. Occasionally, there are a few symptoms like these. Left untreated, once dipstick-positive proteinuria appears, end-stage renal disease will develop in 5–10 years.

The development of diabetic nephropathy in type II diabetes is less well understood. Microalbuminuria itself shows a higher risk of death from heart attack or stroke. How albumin in the urine—when a person has normal kidney function—causes more macrovascular deaths is not known. However, the more albumin in the urine, the higher the rise in cholesterol levels.

Without treatment, after 10 years, about 80 percent of people with type II diabetes and dipstick-positive proteinuria die of heart attack or stroke. For groups of people who are likely to develop type II diabetes, such as the Pima Indians, diabetic nephropathy occurs about as often as it does in people with type I diabetes (or 30–50 percent of these people will get it after having diabetes for 40 years).

Two Major Lines of Defense

Because of new research, doctors now have information to help prevent and treat diabetic nephropathy, and the outlook will likely improve. As with other medical conditions, treatments are much more effective when they are started early. It's crucial to avoid damage to the kidneys if at all possible. Controlling both your blood glucose levels and blood pressure levels can help.

Blood glucose control

Excellent blood glucose control will help prevent nephropathy. In the DCCT, the tight blood glucose control of the intensive therapy group decreased their risk of developing microalbuminuria by 35 percent. It decreased clinical nephropathy by 56 percent. Although all the people in this trial had type I diabetes, other studies have reported the same benefits for people with type II diabetes.

If people have protein in the urine, the effect of various treatments will depend on how advanced the kidney disease is. In people with type I diabetes and microalbuminuria (but no hypertension), most studies show that improving blood glucose control causes the amount of albumin in the urine to either level off or decrease. Eating a smaller amount of protein daily also seems to help slow diabetic nephropathy. (Although most Americans eat more protein than necessary, a dietitian should help you make this adjustment to your meal plan.)

Blood pressure control

In type I diabetes, it is rare for people to have high blood pressure unless there is already some protein in the urine (proteinuria). However, in type II diabetes, high blood pressure is quite common, with or without kidney disease. One of the most important parts of treatment of diabetic nephropathy is blood pressure control. This is true for those with microalbuminuria or clinical nephropathy. In fact, treatment of high blood pressure at the microalbuminuria stage may stop the nephropathy from getting worse in some people.

The recommended goal for blood pressure in a person with diabetic nephropathy is 120–130/80–85 mmHg. These goals may not be possible for elderly people. The blood pressure of many older people falls to very low levels when they stand. If they try to reach "normal" blood pressure, which is measured while they are sitting, they may have dangerously low blood pressure when they stand. Some become dizzy; others may pass out.

How to Keep Hypertension at Bay

Many studies show that a group of blood pressure medications called angiotensin-converting enzyme inhibitors (ACEIs) slow the development of diabetic nephropathy— even when blood pressure is normal. ACEIs appear to lower microalbuminuria and keep the kidneys working. Many ACEIs are available (Table 8–1). Although there are some differences between the drugs, scientists believe that they all help with diabetic nephropathy in the same way. It appears that the part of the kidney where the blood is filtered, the glomerulus, has too high a pressure in people with diabetic nephropathy (Figure 8–1). Most researchers believe this is the main problem of diabetic nephropathy. ACEIs lower this pressure, which results in less protein leaking from the blood into the urine.

Side effects of ACEIs

The most common side effect from the ACEIs is a cough. This is often described as a tickle in the throat, and,

Table 8-1
Angiotensin-Converting Enzyme Inhibitors

Generic Name	Trade Name
Benazapril	Lotensin
Captopril	Capoten
Enalapril	Vasotec
Fosinopril	Monopril
Lisinopril	Prinivil, Zestril
Moexipril	Univasc
Quinapril	Accupril
Ramipril	Altace

although it's usually just a nuisance, it may get so bad that the drug can't be used. If a person coughs using one ACEI, use of a different one may improve the problem. The other possible problem is that ACEIs may increase the potassium level in the blood. This is more common in older people or those with poor kidney function.

Advantages of ACEIs

ACEIs are considered the most important type of blood pressure drug, because they slow kidney disease. They are especially important for people with type I diabetes and more advanced nephropathy (more than 500 mg of protein in the urine each day, with the kidney functioning only at 40–90 percent of normal). One study reported that the drug captopril can lower the risk of death, dialysis, or transplantation by 50 percent after 3 years of treatment. Other studies have reported the same effects. The Food and Drug Administration has approved captopril for the treatment

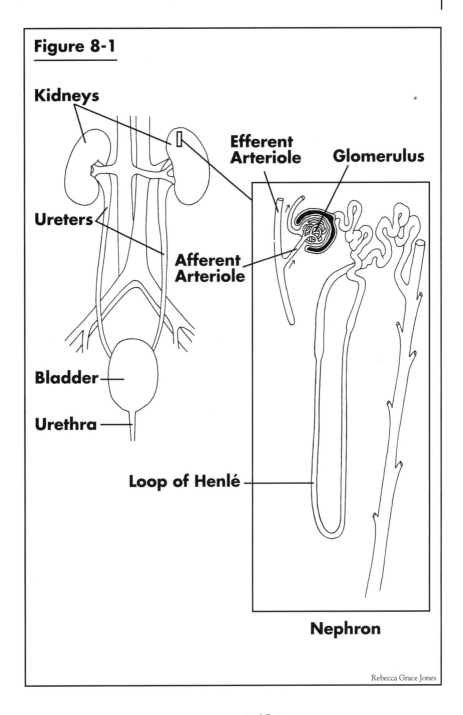

Figure 8-1

Kidneys

Ureters

Bladder

Urethra

Efferent Arteriole

Glomerulus

Afferent Arteriole

Loop of Henlé

Nephron

Rebecca Grace Jones

of diabetic nephropathy in people with type I diabetes and more than 500 mg of proteinuria each day.

Who can't use ACEIs

Some people with impaired kidney function may take an ACEI, and their kidneys may get worse. An ACEI may also lead to high potassium levels in the blood. This is why you must have blood tests to measure creatinine (a measure of kidney function) and potassium soon after starting treatment. In addition, ACEIs may not be used in pregnant women, because they may seriously harm the baby.

Dealing With Other Health Problems

Besides blood glucose levels and blood pressure, other health problems must be considered. First, urinary tract infections need to be treated quickly and well. This means checking a urine culture after the infection has been treated to be sure that the infection is completely gone.

Medications to avoid

Drugs that could harm kidney function should be avoided. These include over-the-counter drugs, such as ibuprofen (Advil, Motrin, and others) and naproxen (Aleve). These are nonsteroidal anti-inflammatory drugs and are called NSAIDs. There are also more than 20 other prescription nonsteroidal anti-inflammatory medications. Fortunately, most drugs that are harmful to the kidneys are either used very seldom or other less harmful drugs can be substituted for them. For example, a class of antibiotics called aminoglycosides are used for serious infections that usually require hospitalization. These drugs can seriously damage the kidneys. For people at risk for nephropathy, doctors can prescribe another antibiotic.

Other antibiotics that can be harmful to the kidneys include

- amphotericin B, used in the treatment of life-threatening fungal infections
- pentamidine, used for people with acquired immunodeficiency syndrome (AIDS)
- cisplatin, used to treat cancer
- acyclovir, used to treat herpes infections; usually harmful to kidneys when taken intravenously but not when taken orally

X rays

Drugs are not the only things that can harm the kidneys. When the dye used for a type of X-ray study is injected into a vein or artery, kidneys can begin to fail in a few days. These dyes, or contrast agents, are used in computed tomography (CT) scans; angiograms, which are commonly used to evaluate the vascular system in people with diabetes; and intravenous pylograms (IVPs), used to evaluate the structure of the kidneys. Although many of these may be replaced with other tests, it is sometimes necessary to use a dye. Fortunately, getting enough fluids intravenously may decrease the risk of kidney damage both before and after the test. Also, a new type of dye is now available that has less potential to damage the kidneys. This new non-ionic contrast dye is much more expensive, however.

Bladder problems

The last problem that might interfere with kidney function is a neurogenic bladder, a bladder that cannot empty

urine normally. Typical symptoms include frequent urination, leaking, and urinary tract infections that keep com-
ing back. Patients with this condition often complain of a
sensation of a full bladder even after voiding. The danger
is that urine in the bladder can back up to the kidneys and
cause kidney damage. There are several strategies your
doctor can use to treat a neurogenic bladder.

What About Testing?

ADA recommends yearly screens for nephropathy in adults
with type II diabetes and in young people past puberty
who have had diabetes for 5 years. The testing may start
with a urine dipstick for proteinuria. If this is positive,
there is probably more than 300 mg of albumin (or 500 mg
of protein) in the urine every day. This needs to be confirmed with a 24-hour urine collection, which would check
for both proteinuria and kidney function.

If the initial dipstick is negative, then a check for microalbuminuria is needed. There are several ways to screen for
microalbuminuria. Doctors frequently order a timed urine
collection, which can be for 24 hours or a shorter period.
Many doctors find it easier to measure the ratio of albumin to creatinine from a random urine specimen. If this
screen for microalbuminuria is negative, the test should be
done yearly. If the screen is positive, it should be confirmed shortly afterward with another screen. If that test
is also positive, treatment should be considered. This may
include starting on an ACEI, even if the person doesn't
have high blood pressure. If hypertension is already being
treated with another drug, switching to an ACEI may be
considered. Better blood glucose control and limiting the

amount of protein in meals may also help at this early stage of nephropathy.

There is much research going on now about diabetic nephropathy. One major question yet to be answered is which genetic and biological abnormalities can cause nephropathy. Researchers are examining whether experimental drugs can slow the progression of nephropathy once it starts. Finally, we need better treatment strategies for people with end-stage renal disease. Statistics from 1994 show that nearly half the diabetic people beginning dialysis die within 2 years, and people receiving a kidney transplant live longer. Heart attacks are the most common cause of

---

Questions to Ask Your Doctor

How does blood glucose control affect my kidneys?
What can I use for a headache or muscle ache if I'm not supposed to use Advil or Aleve?
What do I do if another doctor wants to take an X ray or do a CT scan?
How often should I be tested for protein in my urine?
What's a good blood pressure goal for me?

Questions Your Doctor May Ask You

Do you have any family members with kidney disease?
When were you diagnosed with diabetes?
Have you had a test for glomerular filtration rate (GFR)?
Did your parents have high blood pressure? Did you have high blood pressure as a child or adolescent?
Are you taking blood pressure medication?
Do you take over-the-counter medicines such as Advil?

death for people with advanced nephropathy. More research is needed on early and late nephropathy.

Remember the results of the DCCT. Bringing your blood glucose levels as close to normal as you can will help prevent or slow the development of kidney disease.

■ 9

Hypertension

Hypertension, or high blood pressure, by itself doesn't usually have symptoms as dramatic as those of eye disease or kidney disease. Nevertheless, it is a serious problem that you should not ignore. Hypertension increases your risk of heart attack, eye problems, and kidney disease.

You can take big steps toward lowering your blood pressure with diet, exercise, and medication, if needed.

What Is High Blood Pressure?

The definition

Blood is pumped from the heart to the rest of the body through arteries, branching out into smaller arterioles, and then reaching the capillary beds, where nutrients and oxygen can be exchanged. Blood pressure is the pressure or tension of the blood within the arteries. The pressure is caused by the pump that is the heart, how elastic the arterial walls are, and the resistance of the arterioles. Blood pressure is typically written as one number over another. The top number, the systolic blood pressure, refers to the maximum blood pressure, which occurs when the heart pumps. The bottom number, the diastolic blood pressure, refers to the minimum blood pressure, which occurs during the relaxation time between heartbeats.

What's normal

Normal blood pressure is 120/80 mmHg. Children's blood pressure is lower, and it rises with age. When blood pressure levels are consistently too high, it's called hypertension. A 1993 consensus panel decided that blood pressure that stays above 140/90 requires therapy. This therapy could include lifestyle changes, medication, or both. It is common for people older than 60 to have higher systolic blood pressure but normal diastolic blood pressure levels. This is because arterial walls become less elastic as they age. Systolic hypertension—as serious a problem as regular hypertension—is a systolic blood pressure above 140 with a diastolic pressure less than 90 mmHg.

Who gets hypertension

An estimated 3 million Americans have both diabetes and hypertension. Things that influence whether you will have hypertension include your sex, race, and age, how long you have had diabetes, and whether you have protein in your urine. Hypertension is more common in people with type II diabetes than in those with type I diabetes. People with type I diabetes generally have hypertension only if they also have kidney disease.

With type II diabetes, 64 percent of people between the ages of 45 and 65 have hypertension. In contrast, only 25 percent of people who do not have diabetes have hypertension. Before age 50, hypertension is more common in men with type II diabetes, and after 50, it is more common in women.

Hypertension is also more common in certain races. For instance, 58 percent of nondiabetic African Americans have hypertension, compared to 37 percent of white people. In people with type II diabetes, however, the contrast is not as great: 63 percent of African Americans and 50 percent of white people have hypertension.

The risk of heart attack and stroke is almost doubled in diabetic people who also have hypertension. Peripheral vascular disease (blocked arteries to the legs and feet) occurs more often if you have both hypertension and diabetes. In addition, hypertension in people with diabetes may make retinopathy worse.

Finally, it also has a direct and damaging connection with kidney disease.

Advantages of Controlling Blood Pressure

It seems reasonable that controlling your blood pressure would benefit all these complications. Surprisingly, there are no studies of the impact of blood pressure control on macrovascular disease (heart attack, stroke, or peripheral vascular disease) in people with diabetes. However, studies of people without diabetes have shown the benefits of lowering blood pressure. Most experts believe the same results occur in people with diabetes. Macrovascular complications of hypertension are much the same in people with or without diabetes, except that they progress faster in people with diabetes.

In the general population, lowering blood pressure lowers the rate of stroke, heart failure, progression of kidney disease, and retinopathy that occurs with hypertension. Hypertensive retinopathy is different from diabetic retinopathy, in both its causes and symptoms.

None of these studies, however, have found a reduction in death rates from heart attack with blood pressure therapy. Possible reasons for this are 1) some of the drugs used and 2) the fact that many of these trials included small numbers of people. It appears that lowering blood pressure may slow the development of diabetic retinopathy. Some researchers believe there may be reason to use ACEIs in people with hypertension and diabetic retinopathy, because they might benefit, but more research is needed. It is well established, however, that controlling blood pressure helps people with diabetic kidney disease.

Treatment Before Drugs

How it's diagnosed

The diagnosis of hypertension should be based on blood pressure measurements taken on at least three occasions. Although this is usually done in a doctor's office, home blood pressure monitoring can be an important tool to help with the diagnosis and treatment of hypertension.

There has been some concern about the accuracy of some blood pressure machines that you can buy in department stores or pharmacies. These devices are not ideal for diagnosing hypertension. However, many people have "white coat hypertension"—their blood pressure is high only in the doctor's office, because of nervousness or anxiety—so keeping track of blood pressure levels outside the doctor's office or clinic is helpful.

Blood pressure goal

Hypertension in the general population is defined as an average blood pressure of 140/90 mmHg. However, ADA recommends that the goal of blood pressure therapy for diabetic people older than 18 (unless they are pregnant) is to keep blood pressure below 130/85. Further reduction may be possible if done with caution and you feel OK with lower pressure. For those with systolic hypertension and systolic blood pressures above 180, the goal is to reduce the systolic blood pressure to below 160. If the initial systolic blood pressure is between 160 and 179, the goal is to reduce it by 20. If you feel OK—no dizziness, especially on standing—it may be all right to reduce the blood pressure even further.

Drug interactions

ADA recognizes that drug therapy for high blood pressure should not make your blood glucose control worse, raise your lipid levels, or aggravate any problems such as peripheral vascular disease, emphysema, or gout. The side effects of some drugs used to treat hypertension may affect one or more of these conditions. Occasionally, the benefits of some of these medications outweigh their side effects, as is discussed later in this chapter.

Nonmedication treatments

Not everyone with hypertension needs medication right away. For mild to moderate hypertension (140–179/90–109 mmHg), lifestyle changes can be tried alone for 3 months before beginning drug therapy. If these changes don't control hypertension, then it's time to turn to drug therapy. For blood pressure above 210/120, however, or if the person has diabetic kidney disease, drug therapy should be started as soon as the hypertension is diagnosed.

Therapy before trying drugs includes
- losing weight
- restricting salt
- stopping smoking
- limiting daily alcohol intake to less than 2 ounces (equal to 8 ounces of wine or 24 ounces of beer)
- doing regular aerobic exercise

All these can improve mild hypertension or lower the risk of a heart attack or stroke. Making all these changes permanent can be difficult, however, and ADA suggests that you have individual counseling with group or peer support to help you.

Drug Treatment

In 1993, ADA published a consensus statement (see Chapter 1) about treating hypertension with drugs. The panel of experts could not reach agreement that, in the absence of diabetic kidney disease, any one class of drugs was best to start treating hypertension. Each class of drugs has advantages and disadvantages. Certain situations, discussed below, may make one class of drug more attractive for specific people.

The drugs are listed in the order that they became available for use in the United States, with the "oldest" drugs discussed first.

Thiazide diuretics

Small doses of thiazide diuretics, such as hydrochlorothiazide at 12.5–25 mg daily, lower blood pressure. In the general population, these drugs lower the risk of death from stroke and congestive heart failure but not from heart attack. The reasons are not clear but may be because of side effects of these drugs. These drugs are particularly helpful in lowering blood pressure in African Americans. Another advantage is that they are inexpensive.

The major disadvantage of this class of drugs is how they affect your blood chemistry. They tend to
- increase blood glucose levels (at least in people with type II diabetes)
- increase lipid levels (triglycerides, total cholesterol, and LDL cholesterol)
- lower potassium and magnesium levels
- increase serum uric acid levels, which may occasionally make gout worse

Fortunately, use of lower doses means fewer side effects. One of the most heated debates in medicine is the role of thiazide diuretics as the first drug used to treat hypertension, particularly in people with diabetes. There is agreement that thiazide diuretics should not be used alone to treat hypertension in people with diabetic nephropathy.

On the other hand, there may be advantages to using thiazide diuretics in people with early diabetic nephropathy who are taking an ACEI. Overall, thiazide diuretics work well in combination with other drugs for hypertension.

ß-Blockers (Beta-Blockers)

These drugs continue to be popular first-line drugs in the treatment of hypertension in the United States. Several ß-blockers have been shown to decrease heart attacks and death rates related to high blood pressure in the general population. After heart attacks, they prevent future heart attacks and sudden death for up to 18 months regardless of whether the person has diabetes.

Many ß-blockers are available, and they may be classified as selective or nonselective (Table 9–1). These drugs, however, may:

- slow the recovery of a hypoglycemic episode
- mask some typical symptoms of low blood glucose (tremor, palpitations, and anxiety) and exaggerate other symptoms (such as sweating)
- worsen blood glucose control for people with type II diabetes (but not type I diabetes)
- raise serum triglycerides while lowering HDL (good) cholesterol
- make peripheral vascular disease worse

All of these side effects may not occur or will occur less often with the selective ß-blockers. So the selective varieties are preferred for people with diabetes.

ß-Blockers may be the right choice—even as the first treatment used—for some people with diabetes. Young people

Table 9–1
ß-Blockers Available in the United States

	Generic Name	Trade Name
Selective	Acebutolol	Sectral
	Atenolol	Tenormin
	Betaxolol	Kerlone
	Bisoprolol	Zebeta
	Metoprolol	Lopressor
		Toprol XL
Nonselective	Carteolol	Cartrol
	Nadolol	Corgard
	Penbutolol	Levatol
	Pindolol	Visken
	Propranolol	Inderal
	Propranolol, extended release	Inderal LA
	Timolol	Blocadren

with a rapid pulse rate seem to respond well to these agents. ß-Blockers may be very useful for people who have chest pain, known as angina, but not heart failure. These drugs are also frequently used to treat high blood pressure during pregnancy.

Angiotensin-converting enzyme inhibitors (ACEIs)
ACEIs are discussed in detail in Chapter 8 (Table 8–1). Besides their beneficial effect in lowering blood pressure, they also slow the progress of diabetic kidney disease, regardless of high blood pressure. These drugs have no bad

effects on lipid levels or blood glucose control. Cough is the most common side effect, and sometimes it is so severe that the drug must be stopped. Potassium levels in the blood can rise to dangerous levels, particularly in people whose kidneys are not working well; so, it should be watched carefully. ACEIs should not be used during pregnancy; women of child-bearing age—who may not know whether they are pregnant—should use them with caution.

Calcium-channel blockers
Besides high blood pressure, these drugs are often used to treat angina. Like ACEIs, they do not change lipid levels or blood glucose control. Both calcium-channel blockers and ACEIs rarely affect sexual function. Thiazide diuretics and ß-blockers, however, can cause difficulty in maintaining an erection.

Several calcium-channel blockers have both short-acting and long-acting forms (See Table 9–2). One may work better for you than another. For example, if short-acting nifedipine needs to be taken three times daily, what happens to your blood pressure if the midday dose is missed three times each week? This is not a concern with a medication taken only once daily. People are more likely to take medication on schedule if they only have to take it once a day.

α-Blockers (Alpha Blockers)
These drugs are as effective as thiazide diuretics, ß-blockers, ACEIs, and calcium-channel blockers for the treatment of high blood pressure (See Table 9-3). They also work well in combination with other drugs. They do not have a bad effect on lipid levels or blood glucose control. The major concern is orthostatic hypotension (a decrease in blood pressure on

{2}

Table 9–2
Calcium-Channel Blockers Available in the United States

Generic Name	Trade Name
Amlodipine	Norvasc
Diltiazem	Cardizem CD
	Dilacor XR
Felodipine	Plendil
Isradipine	DynaCirc
Nicardipine	Cardene
Nifedipine*	Procardia XL
	Adalat CC
Nislodipine	Sular
Verapamil*	Calan SR
	Isoptin SR
	Verelan

*extended release preparations

standing), which can be so severe that it causes dizziness or even unconsciousness. This side effect is less common with doxazocin than prazocin. Doxazocin and terazosin are also approved for the treatment of benign prostatic hypertrophy, a noncancerous enlargement of the prostate, and so may be a particularly good choice for older men.

Factors to Consider

Differences among drugs
Overall, there are small differences among drugs in each group. For example, enalapril, lisinopril, and captopril—

Table 9–3
α-Blockers Available in the United States

Generic Name	Trade Name
Doxazocin	Cardura
Prazosin	Minipress
Terazosin	Hytrin

all ACEIs—decrease blood pressure levels and reduce protein in the urine in people with diabetic kidney disease. However, their side effects are different. For example, skin rash is more common with captopril.

Calcium-channel blockers (Table 9–2) have important differences. For instance, verapamil tends to slow the heart rate and may cause constipation, while nifedipine generally does not affect heart rate or bowel habits. Some studies have shown that proteinuria increases with nifedipine but it decreases with diltiazem.

One size doesn't fit all

The blood pressure medications discussed in this chapter are not a complete list. Like many other parts of diabetes therapy, the treatment of high blood pressure isn't like a cookbook, where you can simply follow the directions. One therapy doesn't work for everyone. Your doctor should regularly review the affects of your lifestyle and any of these drugs you may be taking. You should also ask your doctor about any nonprescription drugs you are taking or thinking about taking. Many medications, including those you can buy over the counter, can raise your blood pressure. Nonsteroidal anti-inflammatory drugs, such as ibuprofen; oral contraceptives; certain antidepressants called tricyclics, such as amitriptyline and nortriptyline; and decongestants, such as pseudoephedrine, may all raise blood pressure.

Consider the costs

Some of the cost of therapy may not be obvious. For example, a person may be treated with a diuretic, which can cause low potassium levels. The potassium level must be watched by the doctor, and often the person will need a potassium supplement or to switch to another drug. The

---

Questions to Ask Your Doctor

How can I find a counselor (dietitian, personal trainer, etc.) to help me lose weight, stop smoking, start exercising, etc.?

Where can I find support groups for losing weight, stopping smoking, stopping or slowing alcohol intake?

How does stress affect my blood pressure? What about coffee?

What if I miss my blood pressure pill? Should I take an extra one later?

Questions Your Doctor May Ask You

Do you take any over-the-counter medications?

What prescription drugs do you take?

Does anyone in your family have hypertension?

What do you do for exercise?

Do you use salt? Do you eat high-salt foods, such as canned soups?

Have you had any side effects from blood pressure medications in the past?

---

diuretic may end up costing more than another drug choice. Generic drugs are usually much cheaper. However, these drugs often have to be taken more than once daily, so they may not be much cheaper. And the disadvantage of taking a drug more than once a day is that you are likely to forget to take it.

Because hypertension is so common in people with diabetes, future research will need to show which drugs are best for preventing heart attack and stroke, with or without diabetic nephropathy.

■ 10

Lipids and Exercise

Lipids are body fats. These include triglycerides and cholesterol. Because one of the best ways to treat lipid problems is physical activity, this chapter covers both topics.

There are several types of lipids or fats. Triglycerides and cholesterol are found in animal foods and are also created by the body. The body uses triglycerides as stored fat to keep you warm, protect your organs, and give you energy. Cholesterol, despite its bad reputation, has many valuable jobs. It is an important part of cell membranes. It is stored in endocrine glands (such as the adrenals, testes, and ovaries) and can be converted to hormones (such as cortisol, testosterone, and estrogen). In the liver, cholesterol helps make bile acids.

Neither triglyceride nor cholesterol can be dissolved in water (or blood). They travel in the blood by joining with proteins that carry them in and out of the body tissues.

These carriers are called lipoproteins, a combination of the words *lipid* and *protein*.

LDL (low-density lipoprotein) is the major carrier for cholesterol in the blood. LDL is called the "bad" cholesterol. When you have too much LDL cholesterol, it sticks to your blood vessel walls and forms plaque, a condition called atherosclerosis. Plaque gets in the way of the blood flowing through an artery. If an artery in the heart has this buildup on its walls, angina or a heart attack may happen. If one of the arteries supplying blood to the brain is blocked by these deposits, a stroke may occur.

HDL (high-density lipoprotein) takes cholesterol away from the blood vessel walls and into the liver, where it is used for other purposes. This is called the "good" cholesterol. Studies have shown that high levels of HDL in your blood lower your risk of a heart attack or stroke.

What Can Go Wrong

Problems arise when your levels of triglycerides and LDL and HDL cholesterol are out of balance. The most common problems in type II diabetes have to do with triglycerides and HDL cholesterol. People with type II diabetes have higher triglyceride levels than the general population, but losing weight will lower these triglyceride levels for both groups. The triglyceride levels need to be lower because the higher the triglyceride level is, the lower the level of HDL cholesterol. Among people with type II diabetes, women tend to have higher HDL cholesterol than men, and African Americans have higher levels than white people.

For people with type I diabetes, ketoacidosis can throw your lipid levels way out of balance. These lipid imbalances start to improve as soon as blood glucose control improves.

Cholesterol

People with type II diabetes have the same total cholesterol and LDL cholesterol levels as people without diabetes who are about the same age and weight. However, this is misleading. The LDL cholesterol in people with type II diabetes is smaller and denser. These small, dense particles are more likely to cause atherosclerosis than the larger LDL cholesterol in nondiabetic people. What helps is to lose weight. This brings triglyceride levels down, and there is less of the dense LDL as well.

LDL cholesterol levels get higher with age, at least up to about age 55 in men and 65 in women. But most important, LDL cholesterol levels are higher in people who eat more saturated fat and cholesterol. (Saturated fats contain cholesterol and raise blood cholesterol levels. Some foods that are high in saturated fat are meat, butter, and eggs.) For example, Americans with type II diabetes have higher LDL cholesterol levels than Japanese with type II diabetes, possibly because the Japanese eat a lower-fat diet. Higher LDL cholesterol levels may be the major reason for differences in the rate of heart disease among different ethnic groups.

Cardiovascular risks

People with type I diabetes with good blood glucose control have about the same lipid levels as the general population. Poor diabetes control in people with type I diabetes means high triglyceride and LDL cholesterol levels, endangering the health of their blood vessels. In all diabetic people with protein in the urine—a sign of kidney disease— the levels of triglyceride and LDL cholesterol go up and that of HDL cholesterol goes down. This appears to be one reason people with diabetic kidney disease have more problems with heart disease and stroke.

Cardiovascular disease damages blood vessels all over the body, not only arteries to the heart, which could result in heart attack. Cerebrovascular disease in the blood vessels to the brain could lead to stroke. Peripheral vascular disease in the blood vessels to the limbs could result in amputation of all or part of a foot or limb. Your risk of cardiovascular disease can be measured by

- high blood pressure
- high total cholesterol
- cigarette smoking

If you have two or more of these risk factors, your chances of having cardiovascular disease are dramatically increased—and people with diabetes already have four to five times the risk of nondiabetic people. Most scientists believe that having both low HDL cholesterol and high triglyceride levels is an added risk for patients with type II diabetes. Also, abdominal obesity, or being shaped like an apple with most of the fat being carried at the belt level instead of at the hips (like a pear), appears to be another risk factor for cardiovascular disease.

When testing should be done

ADA recommends that children with diabetes who are more than 2 years old have a lipid profile done both after diagnosis and when glucose control has improved. If the results fall within acceptable levels (Table 10–1), the test should be repeated every 5 years. Yearly testing is recommended for children whose results are too high.

Adults with high or out-of-balance lipids should be tested each year for total cholesterol, fasting triglycerides, and HDL and LDL cholesterol. If treatment (including diet and exercise) is started, repeat the tests as needed to see how the treatment is working. When all levels are in the acceptable range, you don't need to be tested so often. If total or LDL cholesterol is high, thyroid-stimulating hormone (TSH) should be measured to check for low thyroid levels. Low thyroid levels are quite common, especially with type I diabetes, and may cause high cholesterol levels.

Treating Lipid Problems

People with poorly controlled diabetes often have high levels of triglycerides, total cholesterol, and LDL cholesterol, and low levels of HDL cholesterol. This imbalance

Table 10–1
Lipid Levels for Adults With Diabetes

Risk	Cholesterol (mg/dl)	HDL Cholesterol (mg/dl)	LDL Cholesterol (mg/dl)	Triglycerides (mg/dl)
Acceptable	<200	—	<130	<200
Borderline	200–239	—	130–159	200–399
High	≥240	<35	≥160	>400

improves when blood glucose levels are more controlled. In the DCCT, lipid levels were healthier in the intensive therapy group (see Chapter 3). The standard therapy group had LDL cholesterol that was denser and more likely to block an artery. That's why the first approach to balancing your lipid levels should be to improve your blood glucose control with better meal planning and exercise.

Weight loss

The first strategy should be weight loss, if needed. Weight loss has many benefits for diabetes, including
- lowering triglyceride levels
- more normal blood glucose levels
- lowering total cholesterol and LDL cholesterol levels
- raising HDL cholesterol levels

Generally, the greater the weight loss, the greater the improvement in all these areas. But even a small weight loss (less than 10 pounds) can bring about better lipid levels. The way to lose weight is to cut back on your total calories and the amount of fat you eat and to increase your physical activity. This results in slow, steady weight loss that is less likely to come back. (Most dietitians recommend losing no more than 1–2 pounds a week.)

Physical activity

Exercise is also a recommended treatment for lipid problems in people with diabetes. Doing more physical activity makes weight loss and keeping the weight off easier. Losing weight lowers triglyceride, total cholesterol, and LDL cholesterol levels and increases HDL cholesterol levels.

Ease into it. It is impossible to give general recommendations for physical activity. Many things need to be considered before you begin an exercise program. If you have been "sitting" for years, you may be in poor physical condition and may have trouble getting started on exercising. People over age 35 who are not already exercising regularly should have a physical exam (including a stress test) before beginning an exercise program. The medical exam should include

- a check of your blood glucose control—the glycated hemoglobin level
- a cardiovascular exam (blood pressure, peripheral pulses, ECG at rest and during exercise for people older than 35 years or with a history of cardiovascular disease)
- a neurological exam
- a dilated eye exam if proliferative retinopathy is present or suspected

Consider the feet. The doctor should check circulation and sensitivity in your feet. People with any sign of a problem should avoid forms of exercise that involve injury to the feet, such as running or kicking. Proper shoes and socks are particularly important for people with diabetes to avoid injuries or stress to the feet.

Beware of weight lifting-type exercises. Most people with diabetes who have active proliferative retinopathy (see Chapter 7) or uncontrolled high blood pressure should avoid high-intensity exercises such as weight lifting done with a bearing-down motion or holding your breath. These types of activities could increase pressure on the retina and cause more bleeding. If you want to lift weights, get instruction from a qualified teacher, and use lighter weights for more repetitions to build strength. Rhythmic exercises such as walking, jogging, swimming, and cycling are better choices.

Monitor carefully to prevent hypoglycemia. If you take insulin or a sulfonylurea, exercise that lasts for more than 20 minutes will make it work better (see Appendix 2). That's why your blood glucose can get too low during exercise or for as long as 12 hours later. SMBG after exercise helps you decide how to adjust your medication to prevent hypoglycemia. You may need to decrease the amount of insulin you take when you exercise. This is particularly important if you are exercising partly to lose weight. You don't want to have to eat to treat low blood glucose that is caused by exercise when one of the reasons you are exercising is to lose weight.

People with type II diabetes that is controlled by diet alone or diet with metformin or acarbose (see Appendix 2), are not at risk for hypoglycemia and do not need snacks during exercise.

What you should eat

Meal planning for treatment of lipid problems in diabetes should include
  • fewer calories for people needing to lose weight
  • less than 30 percent of daily calories from fat of all kinds
  • less than 10 percent of daily calories from saturated fat
  • less than 300 mg of cholesterol per day

Guidelines to Safe Exercise

- Carry an identification card and wear a bracelet, necklace, or tag at all times that identifies you as having diabetes.

If you use insulin:
- Avoid exercise when your insulin is working hardest (its peak action time) (see Appendix 2).
- Don't inject insulin in an arm or a leg you'll be exercising, because activity will increase the blood flow and cause the insulin to be absorbed faster than usual.
- Your insulin dose may need to be decreased. Check with your health care team about making adjustments for your needs.

For type I diabetes, decreasing insulin by 20 percent before exercise is usually enough to prevent hypoglycemia. For longer activity (such as long-distance cycling or backpacking), a decrease in total insulin dose by 30–50 percent may be necessary.

For type II diabetes, if only one injection of intermediate-acting insulin is usually given (NPH or Lente), decrease the dose by 30 percent. Or, it may be easier to shift to two or more injections per day, with or without adding short-acting insulin. If a combination of intermediate-acting and short-acting insulin is used, both doses may be decreased by up to 30 percent. Check with your health care team for the best ways to do this.
- Be alert for the signs of hypoglycemia during and for up to 12 hours after exercise. Sometimes exercise will affect your blood glucose the next day.
- Always carry a source of carbohydrate (such as glucose tablets) to treat hypoglycemia.
- If your fasting blood glucose is above 300 mg/dl before you exercise, do not exercise until your glucose is below 240 mg/dl and under control.
- Drink fluids before, after, and, if necessary, during exercise to prevent dehydration.

- 50–60 percent of daily calories from carbohydrates. Carbohydrates are found in grains, cereals, breads, pastas, beans, starchy vegetables, milk products, and fruits. Carbohydrates raise blood glucose and are important in a healthy diet for anyone, with or without diabetes.
- daily servings of soluble fiber (beans, oats, and some fruits and vegetables). Fiber may help lower blood glucose and may have beneficial effects on total cholesterol and LDL cholesterol.

Medication

When meal planning, exercise, and glucose control do not control lipid levels, ADA has recommendations for starting therapy with a specific lipid-lowering drug. Treatment with drugs is recommended when a person has one of the following:

- LDL cholesterol remaining above 160 mg/dl
- triglycerides above 400 mg/dl for 6 months (Table 10–1).

Other factors pointing to a lipid-lowering agent are

- HDL cholesterol below 35 mg/dl
- cigarette smoking
- hypertension
- a family history of premature heart disease (before age 60 in men and 70 in women)

The guidelines for lipid levels are even stricter if you have cardiovascular disease. These high-risk people need to have an LDL cholesterol below 100 mg/dl and triglycerides below 200 mg/dl. These guidelines are based on studies of people who do not have diabetes.

There are no specific studies of the effects of lipid-lowering medications on heart attack and stroke in people with diabetes. Studies that have included people with diabetes are relatively short with small numbers of people.

In type II diabetes, high triglyceride levels and low HDL cholesterol levels are common. What should you do when improved diabetes control does not bring the lipid levels back to normal? Drugs used with type II diabetes that improve insulin resistance often lower the triglyceride levels, too. In 1995, the first of these drugs, metformin, was introduced in the United States. Metformin (Glucophage), lowers triglyceride levels by about 16 percent. Other drugs that improve insulin resistance (also called insulin sensitizers) will likely be available soon and have a beneficial effect on triglyceride levels.

The following types of drugs are used to treat problems with lipids (Table 10–2).

Bile acid–binding resins

The two drugs in this class, cholestyramine and colestipol, lower total and LDL cholesterol but don't do much to HDL cholesterol. These drugs help reduce heart disease when used alone or with other drugs. Unfortunately, the bile acid–binding resins may raise triglyceride levels, particularly if those levels are already above 250 mg/dl. That is why these drugs may be difficult for the majority of people with type II diabetes to use. These agents are usually used in small doses and added to other drug therapy.

Table 10–2
Lipid Lowering Agents

	Generic Name	Trade Name
Bile acid–binding resins	Cholestyramine	Questran
	Colestipol	Colestid
Fibric acid derivatives	Gemfibrozil	Lopid
HMG-CoA reductase		
inhibitors	Fluvastatin	Lescol
	Lovastatin	Mevacor
	Pravastatin	Pravachol
	Simvastatin	Zocor
Nicotinic acid	Niacin	Niacor

Neither of these drugs affects blood glucose control, and both may cause problems with constipation.

Fibric acid derivatives
These drugs include gemfibrozil and clofibrate. They lower triglyceride levels and raise HDL cholesterol levels. They are often used by people with type II diabetes. For people with both elevated LDL cholesterol and triglycerides, the fibric acid derivatives work quite well with bile acid–binding resins. Neither gemfibrozil nor clofibrate affects blood glucose, but both may increase the risk of gallstones.

HMG-CoA reductase inhibitors
Also called statins, there are four of these drugs available in the United States. They lower LDL cholesterol levels by 20–35 percent. They do not affect glucose control.

Nicotinic acid

This drug reduces LDL cholesterol and triglycerides and increases HDL cholesterol levels. It is very inexpensive and could be an ideal medication. Unfortunately, it also increases insulin resistance and raises both fasting and after-meal glucose levels. It cannot be a routine medication for people with diabetes.

Estrogen

Before menopause, women without diabetes have a lower risk for cardiovascular disease than men of the same age—possibly because of higher estrogen levels. For various reasons, women with diabetes lose this protection and, after menopause, are at high risk for cardiovascular disease. Most scientists now recommend estrogen therapy for women with diabetes because it will raise HDL cholesterol and reduce their risk. Progestin, which protects against endometrial cancer, should also be given to all women taking estrogen, unless they have had a hysterectomy. In high doses, estrogen may increase triglyceride levels, so lower doses may be given to women with type II diabetes. Some studies suggest that an estrogen patch does not affect triglyceride levels as much as estrogen taken orally.

Aspirin

There is growing enthusiasm about using aspirin as a way to prevent and to treat atherosclerosis. This is because people with diabetes have stickier platelets (the blood cells that start clots). Without platelets—or if they don't work—severe bleeding can occur. On the other hand, blood that clots too quickly because of platelet clumping may add to heart disease and stroke in people with diabetes.

Aspirin, even in very low doses (one baby aspirin each day), can make the platelets less sticky and may lower your risk for atherosclerosis. Indeed, in a meta-analysis (a tool that looks at many studies together to help answer a question) of 145 studies published in 1994, people with diabetes and atherosclerosis who were on aspirin therapy had less risk of death, heart attack, and stroke. Another large study found a 25 percent risk reduction of heart attack with aspirin therapy.

Questions to Ask Your Doctor

Should I be taking aspirin?

What type of exercise should I do?

How can I lower my cholesterol without medication?

If I need medication, what kind is right for me?

Why should I worry about heart disease if no one in my family has it?

How does fish oil affect my cholesterol and triglycerides?

How does smoking affect my cholesterol?

Questions Your Doctor May Ask You

Do you smoke?

Do you have family members with heart disease?

When was your last ECG? Last stress test?

What type of shoes do you wear when you exercise?

Do you ever get chest pain?

Do you ever get shortness of breath?

Do these symptoms occur with exercise?

Does aspirin upset your stomach?

Do you get pain in your calves when you walk?

Do your feet often get cold?

Also, aspirin does not affect diabetic retinopathy. It does not cause further bleeding from the retinopathy. Most researchers now recommend low-dose aspirin (one baby aspirin or one adult aspirin daily) for most people with diabetes. Aspirin is not recommended for people who cannot tolerate the drug (because of stomach pain, stomach ulcer, or allergy) or who have uncontrolled hypertension.

Unanswered questions

Unfortunately, many questions about atherosclerosis and lipid-lowering therapy for people with diabetes are still unanswered. There have not been any large trials with diabetic people specifically addressing this issue. This not only includes drug therapy but also nutrition therapy, particularly in high-risk groups with an even higher risk for heart disease or stroke (for example, people with diabetic kidney disease). Another question that needs an answer is whether postmenopausal women with diabetes benefit more from estrogen therapy than the general population. Finally, we need better ways to treat low levels of HDL cholesterol. This could include lifestyle changes or possibly drug therapy.

■ 11

Diabetic Neuropathy

Diabetic neuropathy is nerve damage caused by too much glucose in your blood over a long period. What goes wrong? Your nerves either can't send messages, send them at the wrong time, or send them too slowly. Symptoms can vary and can include pain in your hands and feet, difficulty digesting food, and bladder and bowel control problems.

The most common type of neuropathy is *peripheral neuropathy*. Peripheral neuropathy may affect different parts of the body, but it usually begins in the feet and legs. Doctors can detect peripheral neuropathy before you notice any symptoms. Unfortunately, complaints about this condition are often what bring people to the doctor in the first place, and then they find out they have diabetes.

Other health problems, however, may have the same symptoms as peripheral neuropathy. These include pernicious anemia (low red blood cell count because of inability to absorb vitamin B$_{12}$ from the stomach), kidney failure, chemical toxins, and neuropathy from alcohol abuse. Alcohol makes diabetic neuropathy worse, so most doctors recommend that people with neuropathy drink little, if any, alcohol. Also, other nerve diseases, such as carpal tunnel syndrome, may be confused with diabetic neuropathy. Your doctor may need to do special electrical stimulation tests of the nerves to make a diagnosis.

Symptoms

Neuropathy can have several different symptoms, including tingling or a pins-and-needles sensation, shooting or stabbing pains, numbness or loss of sensation, or weakness. Touching things such as bedsheets and clothing may be painful. The pain is often worse at night, and many people complain of having trouble falling asleep. The pain usually goes away over time, but it may hang on for years.

The most dangerous symptom of neuropathy is numbness of the feet. Because you can't feel pain, you won't notice when you hurt yourself or develop an infection. For example, if you step on a sharp object such as a piece of glass or have a small pebble inside your shoe, you won't feel it. You may get a large cut, an abrasion, or an ulcer (a deep wound often with dying tissue beneath the surface), and it may get infected. This is why people with neuropathy, especially with numb feet, are at such a high risk for a foot ulcer. These ulcers are called neuropathic foot ulcers, because they result from neuropathy. When these foot ulcers are not treated, they can become infected. The infected foot ulcers can cause a bone infection known as osteomyelitis, which is difficult to treat and can lead to amputation of one or more toes or an entire leg up to the knee.

Who's at Risk

The risks for developing peripheral neuropathy are
- height (taller people have a greater risk)
- sex (more likely to occur in males)
- age (the risk increases as you get older)
- hypertension
- length of time you've had diabetes
- poor glucose control
- high total cholesterol
- smoking

Three-Part Care

Treatment of neuropathy can be divided into three parts: education, treatment of pain, and direct foot care.

The first step is to identify the high-risk foot—the one that may develop a neuropathic foot ulcer. This is important because many people do not feel pain. Doctors should examine your feet at every visit, including checking for calluses, cracks, and other sores. Testing for sensation with the nylon monofilaments (see Chapter 4) is perhaps the best way to check whether you are at risk for a neuropathic foot ulcer.

Education
You and your shoes. If you have a high-risk foot, you and your family need to be taught how to prevent injury. One cause of problems is poor-fitting shoes. Your shoes should

fit well and not make red areas on your feet from rubbing or slipping. The skin in these areas can break down and get infected. If you change your shoes several times a day, you can prevent this from happening. Many doctors suggest that you wear walking or running shoes every day, because they cushion your feet with extra padding. It is no surprise that dress shoes can cause problems, so proper fit is very important. Soft leather shoes are helpful. If your shoes do not fit well, orthotics—specially made devices that support your foot within your shoes—may help. It is important to check your shoes and shake them out before putting them on to make sure there are no objects inside.

Daily foot care. How to take care of your feet is another important part of your education. Feet should be washed daily with mild soap, rinsed, and dried thoroughly, including between the toes. Moisture-restoring creams, especially for dry feet, should be applied once or twice daily but not between the toes (wet areas between the toes increase the risk of developing infection). Always wear socks, and trim your nails with a slightly rounded edge. Do not do any foot "surgery," especially for ingrown toenails, on yourself. See a qualified professional for this care. Many people who cannot see well or who cannot easily reach their own toes prevent problems by having their nails trimmed by a health care provider.

Avoid heating pads. Because you can't determine when it's too hot, heating pads, space heaters, or stoves can cause serious burns that can become infected. Perhaps most important, never go barefoot, even to walk to the bathroom from the bedroom.

Treatment of pain

Unfortunately, no single drug works for everyone who has pain from neuropathy. Some people, especially those whose greatest pain comes from objects that don't usually cause pain (clothing or bedding), find relief with capsaicin cream (Zostrix-HP and Dolorac). This cream is applied four times daily in small amounts on the surface of the sensitive foot.

Some antidepressants, used in smaller doses than for depression, may help, especially when it is a pins-and-needles pain. The most commonly used antidepressants include amitriptyline (Elavil), imipramine (Tofranil), and nortriptyline (Pamelor). Often, doses ranging from 10 to 50 mg daily help relieve the pain from neuropathy. Some people have found fluoxitine (Prozac) helpful, although there are no clinical studies supporting this. Others find help from antiseizure drugs, such as carbamazepine (Tegretol) and phentoin (Dilantin). Several studies have shown that people get relief from mexilitine (Mexitil), a medication used for cardiac arrhythmias (irregular heartbeat). This drug may cause cardiac arrhythmias, however, so it must be used with caution, especially in people who already have this problem.

Direct foot care

The final important treatment is direct foot care with attention focused on problems that increase the risk of amputation.

Calluses. Thick calluses can increase pressure on a specific area by 30 percent. This pressure raises the chance of skin breakdown, so it is wise to reduce the size of the callus. A podiatrist or doctor familiar with the problem should do this. Planing consists of using a brush or sandpaper to sand off part of the callus. Debriding is removal of dead tissue, often with a probe or scalpel. You can use pumice stones gently to help keep smaller calluses under control. Cushioned shoes and pressure-reducing hosiery can also help keep a callus small. If you're getting calluses, it's a clue that you need different shoes or corrective footwear. You may need to be referred to an orthopod, a surgeon specializing in bone diseases, or to a pedorthist, who has been trained to fit shoes properly.

Ulcers. An ulcer is a serious condition that must be seen by the doctor. Because it can take a long time to heal or even lead to amputation, never try to treat one yourself. If the ulcer is infected, as it often is, the infection needs to be treated with antibiotics. Occasionally, the antibiotics will be given through your veins and you may need to be hospitalized. Many of these ulcers will not heal, because severe peripheral vascular disease won't allow enough blood to reach the ulcer. In this case, you may be referred to a vascular surgeon. Angioplasty—in which a balloon is inserted into the blocked blood vessel to move the blockage and allow an increase in blood flow—or bypass surgery may improve blood flow to the foot.

Keep weight off the foot. Whether the ulcer is infected or not, don't walk on it. The healing process is slowed every time you take a step on an ulcer on the bottom of your foot. Although there are several ways to keep your weight off the foot, perhaps the best is a special walking cast or bed rest. The dead tissue should be removed regularly by a health professional. There are several creams and ointments that promote skin and tissue growth, and your doctor could recommend one.

Charcot's joint. A serious complication of the numb foot is diabetic neuroarthropathy, also called Charcot's joint. This often begins with an injury, such as twisting an ankle. Because of loss of feeling in the foot, the person does not feel pain and continues to walk on the injured foot. Often,

Education to Prevent Foot Ulcers

Shoes
Wear well-fitting shoes even if you think they are ugly.
Change shoes during the day to take pressure off sensitive areas.
Try running or walking shoes for everyday wear.
Select dress shoes of soft leather and have them fitted carefully.
Use orthotics to solve fitting problems.
Break in new shoes slowly.
Shake shoes out and inspect them before putting them on for areas that might cause blisters or rubbing.

Foot Hygiene
Wash feet daily with mild soap; rinse and dry thoroughly, especially between the toes.
Apply moisture creams once or twice daily, except between the toes.
Trim nails to have a slightly rounded edge.
Avoid "bathroom self-surgery" and have a qualified professional treat all foot problems.
Do not soak your feet.
Do not use heating pads or sleep next to space heaters or stoves.
Never go barefoot.

Problems to Report Immediately to Your Doctor
Cuts or breaks in the skin
Ingrown nails
Change in color or discoloration of the foot
Change in shape of the foot

the ankle and foot become red and swollen, but because of neuropathy, it does not hurt. At this point, the foot may be infected, even though there are no other clues that infection is present (such as fever). Eventually, the bone will break down. The foot arch is often lost, and eventually the foot becomes so deformed that walking is difficult. Special footwear is very important for Charcot's joint.

Another Type of Neuropathy

Another important type of nerve damage is *autonomic neuropathy*. This is less common than peripheral neuropathy but just as serious. Antonomic neuropathy is damage to the nerves that control parts of the body without you having to think about them. These nerves are more closely involved with the central nervous system (the brain and spinal cord).

Cardiovascular autonomic neuropathy

The earliest sign of cardiovascular autonomic neuropathy is an increase in your heart rate, particularly during sleep, when heart rates are normally quite low. Usually, your heart rate varies with breathing. When you breathe in, heart rate goes up; when you breathe out, heart rate goes down. When autonomic neuropathy affects your heart, the heart rate does not change as you breathe. This type of autonomic neuropathy interferes with the usual symptoms of heart attack. Instead of the sharp chest pain often felt, people with neuropathy may have no symptoms or a mild symptom that they dismiss as indigestion.

Another symptom of cardiovascular autonomic neuropathy is low blood pressure that occurs when you stand up

Symptoms of Autonomic Neuropathy

Cardiovascular autonomic neuropathy (affecting the heart and blood pressure)
- fast resting heart rate
- difficulty exercising
- painless heart attack
- orthostatic hypotension (low blood pressure when the person stands up)

Gastrointestinal autonomic neuropathy
- feeling of esophagus being blocked
- gastroparesis—food stays too long in the stomach
- constipation and/or diarrhea
- leaking of feces

Genitourinary autonomic neuropathy
- neurogenic bladder
- sexual dysfunction (both men and women)

Sudomotor autonomic neuropathy (abnormal sweating)
- facial sweating
- can't tolerate heat
- gustatory sweating (sweating while eating)

Hypoglycemia-associated autonomic failure
- loss of symptoms of hypoglycemia

(orthostatic hypotension). This can be quite difficult to treat. The following will help:
- improved diabetes control
- wearing elastic stockings, which help keep blood in the vascular system
- increased salt intake, which causes water retention and keeps blood pressure up

- medications such as fludrocortisone (Florinef), which cause the kidneys to reabsorb more sodium (salt) and water with it

Gastrointestinal autonomic neuropathy

Gastrointestinal neuropathy affects nerves in the stomach and intestines. When the esophagus (the tube between the mouth and the stomach) does not move food properly, it feels as if the food is "stuck," which can be extremely uncomfortable.

Gastroparesis. Another problem is gastroparesis, which can delay the absorption of food. People with this often have bloating, a feeling of fullness after eating a small meal (or even just a few bites), nausea, and vomiting. Often, the stomach contains undigested food eaten many hours earlier. Besides being uncomfortable, this condition causes a problem with the insulin that was injected before the meal. The food is not being processed on time. The insulin still peaks normally, but the food hasn't yet raised your blood glucose. The result is hypoglycemia, usually after the meal, when the short-acting insulin is working the hardest.

To treat this problem, you should eat small meals that are low in fat and fiber, which are more easily digested. Metoclopromide (Reglan) and cisapride (Propulsid) are used to treat gastroparesis. Some studies have also shown that gastroparesis can be helped with the antibiotic erythromycin as well.

Colon difficulties. Gastrointestinal neuropathy may affect the colon. Constipation alternating with diarrhea is the result. Choosing foods that have lots of insoluble fiber and taking 1–3 tablespoons per day of psyllium will help in most cases. Your doctor may recommend a laxative, such as milk of magnesia, for severe symptoms. For diarrhea, several different things may work. A mixture of kaolin and pectin is often tried first. Later, other drugs such as cholestyramine, antibiotics (tetracycline), loperimide (Imodium), or clonidine may be tried. Octreotide (Sandostatin) is for diarrhea that won't respond to other drugs.

Genitourinary autonomic neuropathy
This includes erection problems, inability to reach orgasm, and neurogenic bladder. A neurogenic bladder has lost feeling—you cannot tell when it is full or whether it has completely emptied. Gradually, you will urinate only once or twice daily. Some people have trouble starting a stream at all. Some people leak urine. Treatment includes timed voiding, double voiding, (urinating several minutes after you have just urinated, to get rid of all the urine), and special muscle exercises. Occasionally, drugs such as bethanechol can be tried. Some people learn to put in a catheter from a doctor or nurse and do it at home when needed.

Impotence is complicated because there is more than one possible cause. Besides neuropathy, impotence may be due to any of the following:
- poor circulation
- blood not staying within the penis during erection
- hormones (low testosterone levels)
- psychological problems

Treatments are available for all of these. When impotence is caused by neuropathy, men may choose to try a vacuum pump; injections of medication that will help maintain an erection, such as alprostadil (Caverject); or a penile implant, which requires surgery.

Abnormal sweating

Usually, the arms and legs sweat very little while the central part of the body has to do extra sweating. In very hot weather, this may lead to heatstroke, because the limbs can't cool off normally. Obviously, it's important to avoid getting overheated. Sweating may also occur when you eat.

Hypoglycemia-associated neuropathy

This condition is an important reason many people do not have the normal warning symptoms—shakiness, heart pounding, anxiousness—of low blood glucose. Epinephrine is the hormone that probably causes most of these symptoms. Having this condition and hypoglycemia may mean you won't have enough epinephrine the next time you have low blood glucose. Early research suggests that, if you avoid hypoglycemia, you may reverse this serious problem.

Conclusion

Each of the diabetic neuropathies can be disabling and difficult to treat. As with all complications, your goal should be prevention. Unfortunately, you may already have neuropathy. As many as 8 percent of people with type II diabetes already have some neuropathy when their diabetes is diagnosed. But bringing your blood glucose under better control will help.

Education is the most important part of therapy, especially for the numb foot. Amputations of the legs or feet can be prevented with proper care. New medications are being tested for the pain but also to prevent the neuropathy from getting worse. Newer medications for gastroparesis, impotence, and other nerve diseases are being tested. In the meantime, and all of the time, the best way to prevent neuropathy is to improve your blood glucose control.

Questions to Ask Your Doctor

Will my numb foot return to feeling normal?
Why is my heart rate fast?
What are the side effects of Reglan? of Cisapride?
What can I do to improve bladder control?
How can I best examine my own feet when I can't see the bottoms?
What do you suggest for the treatment of athlete's foot?
What are the possible treatments for impotence?
Can neuropathy affect my ability to have orgasms or enjoy sex? What can be done?

Questions Your Doctor May Ask You

Do you feel bloated after eating?
Are you often nauseated?
Have you ever had an ulcer or infection on your foot?
Who cuts your toenails?
Do you wear special shoes because of your neuropathy?
Do you break out in a sweat when eating?
Do you run or cause any kind of foot trauma when you exercise?
Do you have frequent constipation alternating with diarrhea?

■ 12

Putting It All Together: Flowcharts, Doctors, and Insurance

Even "routine" diabetes management can be complicated. There is so much that needs to be done! How can you and your doctor remember how often you need your glycated hemoglobin measured, and just when was that last visit to the eye doctor? What were the exact levels recommended for LDL cholesterol and blood pressure, especially when there's proteinuria? When was the protein in the urine last measured? Come to think of it, when was the last time you visited a dietitian?

Using a Flowchart

No one can recall all of this information, including doctors, who may be seeing hundreds of patients. There are a variety of tools available to help everyone involved get this information. Perhaps the best of these tools is the flowchart. Flowcharts, such as the one on pages 148–150, remind both patients and doctors that a particular test needs to be done. Recommended results for these tests (for example, glycated hemoglobin levels) are often included on the flowchart. There should be space for marking the results of the test or simply checking that something was done (for example, a referral to the ophthalmologist).

It's not a surprise that these flowcharts are becoming more sophisticated. For examples, some large clinics (university based and HMOs) have developed a flowchart with "reminders" to the doctor to be sure a particular test will be done. For example, a 50-year-old woman on no medications visits her doctor for a routine appointment. A computer prints out a flowchart that shows her last Pap smear was 18 months ago. In addition, her last mammogram was 9 months ago, her last tetanus booster was 4 years ago, and her cholesterol has never been measured. For this patient, the doctor orders a Pap smear and cholesterol test.

Although these computer lists are becoming more common, most doctors rely on their own flowcharts. To make this simple, ADA has developed a flowchart for doctors and patients to help track diabetes-related needs.

The flowchart on pages 148–150 includes all ADA Clinical Practice Recommendations from 1995. Different guidelines for care are listed in the first column and the ADA standard or frequency in the next. Obviously, the flowchart needs to be updated as recommendations change. This flowchart does not include non-diabetes-related issues (prostate evaluation, mammogram, etc.). Although this flowchart may be included with your medical record, you may find it useful to have your own copy, too.

Are Doctors Following the Standards?

From the surveys taken so far, we have to say no, most doctors are not following the standards. Your greatest concern may be whether the doctor knows about the ADA Clinical Practice Recommendations. What should you do if a doctor tells you that blood glucose control and SMBG are not important? What if the doctor has never examined your feet? What if your insurance will not pay for blood glucose monitoring strips or meal-planning instruction, let alone expensive medications to lower cholesterol or blood pressure?

These are real concerns. Numerous studies have shown that doctors do not generally follow the ADA Clinical Practice Recommendations. For example, in 1993, a survey from the National Institutes of Health (NIH) reported that "primary-care doctors are not fully aware of recommended criteria for intensive treatment of blood glucose in insulin-dependent diabetes." Other surveys have reported that fewer than half of the people with type I and a much smaller number of people with type II diabetes check their blood glucose. A 1995 study of 97,000 people with diabetes (mostly type II) reported that, in 1 year, only 16 percent had even one glycated hemoglobin test, and only 46 percent received an eye exam. A report from Indiana in 1994 reported that only 43 percent of doctors assessed foot sensation, and only 27 percent of patients with diabetes were referred for eye exams. There are countless other examples.

The reasons for these disappointing results are not clear, but one may be that diabetes training in medical school is

Diabetes Continuing Care Checklist*

Factors of Care	ADA Standard/ Frequency	Patient Goals	Goal Reached?
Height			☐
Weight			☐
Diabetes control			
a. Hypoglycemic episodes			☐
• mild (#/month)			☐
• needing assistance (#/month)			☐
b. Hyperglycemic symptoms/ketonuria			☐
c. Current diabetes medication	as needed for diabetes control		☐
• oral agents			☐
• insulin			☐
d. Other current medication			☐
• BP medication			☐
• lipid lowering medication			☐
e. SMBG	as needed for diabetes control		☐
• preprandial glucose	80–120 mg/dl		☐
• bedtime glucose	100–140 mg/dl		☐
• technique check	yearly		☐
f. HbA₁c	< 7%; individualize for patient; type I, every 3 months; type II, as needed		☐

*Adapted from the Diabetes Continuing Care Record, a part of the Diabetes Control Network, a patient education and diabetes management program of ADA and Pfizer, Inc.

Diabetes Continuing Care Checklist*, cont'd

Factors of Care	ADA Standard/ Frequency	Patient Goals	Goal Reached?
Cardiovascular assessment			
a. Pulse rate			☐
b. Blood pressure	<130/85 mmHg		☐
c. Lipid profile	Yearly test if abnormal		☐
• LDL	<130 mg/dl		☐
• HDL	>35 mg/dl males; >45 mg/dl females		
• TG	<200 mg/dl		☐
d. ECG	In adults, baseline and then as needed		☐
Complications*			☐
a. Retinopathy	Yearly dilated eye and visual exam		☐
• Funduscopy	(pts with diabetes >5 yr, age >30 yr, or		☐
• Eye doctor	symptoms or abnormalities		☐
b. Nephropathy			☐
• urinalysis	Yearly		☐
• urine (micro-/albumin)	Yearly		☐
• creatinine/CrCl			☐
c. Neuropathy			☐
• peripheral sensory evaluation			☐
• autonomic			☐

*Adapted from the Diabetes Continuing Care Record, a part of the Diabetes Control Network, a patient education and diabetes management program of ADA and Pfizer, Inc.

Diabetes Continuing Care Checklist*, cont'd

Factors of Care	ADA Standard/ Frequency	Patient Goals	Goal Reached?
d. Vascular			☐
• pulses/bruits			☐
e. Feet (skin, wounds, infection)			☐
f. Oral/periodontal			☐
Lifestyle†			
a. Exercise	20–45 minutes, 3 days a week		☐
b. Smoking	No		☐
c. Stress (job, family, other)	Counseling		☐
d. Adherence	Patient education		☐
• diet			☐
• exercise			☐
• medications			☐
• SMBG			☐
• appointments			☐
e. Continuing diabetes education			☐
f. Continuing nutrition education			☐

†Special attention, referral to specialist, or counseling may be necessary

*Adapted from the Diabetes Continuing Care Record, a part of the Diabetes Control Network, a patient education and diabetes management program of ADA and Pfizer, Inc.

limited. For a condition that is so complex, but so common, you might expect large amounts of time would be given to diabetes training. Unfortunately, there is no standard medical school course for diabetes.

Another reason for the disappointing results could be that it is very difficult to get new information to the practicing doctor after he or she finishes school. Much of the continuing medical education that doctors must attend by law is sponsored by pharmaceutical or drug companies. Doctors obtain much new information from pharmaceutical company representatives who visit their offices. This information could be biased toward using the products of the drug company. Also, if a doctor attends only conferences sponsored by the pharmaceutical company to learn about new (often expensive) medications, he or she does not get further education about other important aspects of diabetes care, such as how to examine feet, the need for referral for a dilated eye exam, or the use of routine aspirin therapy.

So how do you find the best diabetes doctor around?

Talk to the doctor

First, you need to discuss what is expected, both from the doctor and from you. You are the most important member of the health care team, but everyone on the team has certain responsibilities. For the doctor, it may mean reviewing the diabetes flowchart at each visit with you and being sure that all of the guidelines are followed in a way that works for you. Your responsibilities are greater; you work with the doctor, nurse, and dietitian to reach your goals for weight loss, blood glucose control, and other important measures. Your role is even more important if your health insurance does not cover paying for the team. Is your doctor now willing and able to work with you?

Go doctor shopping

For various reasons, you may need to find a different doctor. This is something many of us do periodically because of a change in insurance or a move to a new city. Finding a new doctor can be done several ways. First, you can get doctors' names from friends, the local ADA chapter, or other sources. Many people decide to see an endocrinologist or diabetologist for diabetes care and continue to see a primary care doctor (usually a general practitioner, an internist, or a family doctor) for nondiabetes-related medical problems. Of course, this may not be possible if there are few endocrinologists in your area. Also, some insurance companies, including HMOs, do not allow these specialists to see patients for routine care.

Making the right choice

Finding the ideal doctor can be a challenge. What is best for you may not be best for someone else. For example, if you are a 20-year-old man with type I diabetes and have an interest in physical activities such as marathon running or mountain climbing, your doctor should know a lot about the effects of physical activity on your diabetes. This includes specific recommendations about your insulin doses and food to eat during and after exercise. On the other hand, if you are a 70-year-old woman with type II diabetes, neuropathy, and arthritis, your doctor should know how your medications may affect your diabetes control, what you can do at home to prevent falls, and how you can prevent or treat osteoporosis.

There are various other ways to help you choose a primary care doctor. For example, it may be helpful to talk to medical or nursing professionals who work in the same office or clinic as the doctor you are interested in. Receptionists can also provide information about which doctors are knowledgeable and popular. After you have narrowed down your choice to two or three, you may want to meet the doctors before committing yourself to one. Some doctors are uncomfortable with this, but it is becoming a more common practice. Meeting the doctor might help prevent having to change doctors later, especially if you don't agree on how to treat your diabetes. This would be an excellent time to discuss the ADA Clinical Practice Recommendations or see how willing the doctor is to refer you to an endocrinologist, if necessary.

Ask about specialties

There are other factors to consider when choosing your primary care doctor. Does the doctor have a specialty? For example, many internists practicing primary care have further training as rheumatologists (arthritis doctors), infectious disease specialists, or even oncologists (cancer doctors). If diabetes is your major problem, having a primary care doctor who is either interested in diabetes or an endocrinologist may be desirable. However, if you have diabetes but also have rheumatoid arthritis, it may be better for you to have a rheumatologist as your primary care doctor.

How about board certification?

Board certification is something else you may want to ask about your doctor. This certifies that the doctor has had a certain amount of training for that specialty and has passed a standardized test. Doctors practicing family medicine, internal medicine, or pediatrics can get board certification. Cardiologists (heart problems), rheumatologists, and endocrinologists require further training after the internal medicine training and can also be board certified. Therefore, a board-certified endocrinologist is certified in both internal medicine and endocrinology. A board-eligible endocrinologist has completed all of the required training but has not yet taken or passed the endocrinology examination.

Who's on call?

It would also be wise to ask who covers ("takes calls") for the doctor when he or she is on vacation or sick and on weekends and evenings. This could be important for many reasons. For example, if your doctor is an endocrinologist and you wear an insulin pump, but none of the on-call doctors are familiar with insulin pumps, who will help you with an emergency with your pump?

Ask about waiting times

Wait times are something else you should consider. This includes the amount of time it takes to see a doctor after you make an appointment. If you're a new patient, you'll have to wait longer for your first appointment than for routine return visits, because the first visit requires a bigger block of time. If you have an unpredictable schedule and need the flexibility to quickly schedule a return appointment, some doctors will not be able to meet your needs, because their wait times for return appointments may be greater than 1 or 2 months.

Wait times also include the amount of time it takes to see the doctor once you arrive at the office or clinic. If a doctor keeps you waiting for more than an hour at every appointment, you may want to consider a different doctor. You can often find out about this before seeing the doctor by talking to the office staff.

You should ask how difficult it is to be seen on the same day if you are sick. This is not a problem for most offices or clinics practicing primary care.

Picking the Right Insurance Plan

For some people, picking the right insurance plan may be most important. Studies show that medical costs for people with diabetes are higher because they visit doctor's offices, hospital outpatient departments, and emergency rooms more often than people without diabetes. People with diabetes are also admitted to the hospital more frequently. One recent study concluded that health care for people with diabetes accounted for almost 12 percent of U.S. health-care costs. Unfortunately, 640,000 Americans with diabetes do not have any form of health-care coverage at all. They do not have routine checkups or help with their blood glucose control and receive their health care in expensive emergency room visits.

There are two general types of insurance: prepaid health plans and fee-for-service insurance. For the first, you and/or your employer pay a fixed premium, and you receive comprehensive health care, from routine office visits to hospitalization. Your cost is lowest if you use the network of participating doctors and hospitals. There is often no deductible to pay or paperwork to do. You also will not be expected to pay out large sums of money for services, so you have better control over your budget should unexpected illness occur. You can see specialists if you are referred to them by your primary care doctor or if the specialist also participates in the prepaid plan. Your choice of hospitals is also limited should you require anything other than emergency hospitalization.

HMOs are the best-known type of prepaid health plan. *Managed care* is another term you may have heard. There are several forms of HMOs.

Prepaid health plans

Staff-model HMOs. These employ doctors who are salaried employees. These HMOs own clinics where their doctors see patients. For specialty services that are used infrequently, the HMO may contract with one or more specialists in private practice in the community. The HMO has a great degree of control over what staff doctors do and don't do and what procedures are allowed and not allowed.

Group-model HMOs. The HMO contracts with an organized group of doctors called a medical group. Most of these medical groups are made up of medical and surgical specialists; therefore, the groups are often referred to as multispecialty medical groups. These doctors are not employees of the HMO. These independent groups may serve members of more than one group-model HMO as well as people with other types of health insurance.

Independent-practice associations (IPAs). In some parts of the country, the IPA model has helped new HMOs compete with more established managed-care organizations. An IPA is a group of doctors in private practice who sign contracts with the IPA to provide care to HMO members. IPAs are owned either by a group of doctors or a single doctor. IPAs help an HMO enter a new city and begin operating within a few months at little expense. The doctors in the IPA are free to care for members of any other type of health plan that contracts with them.

Fee-for-service (FFS) insurance

This is the traditional type of health insurance. You and/or your employer pay the insurance company a premium each month. The insurance company agrees to pay for all or some of the medical care you receive. In this pay-as-you-go system, the insurer pays for the service you receive from your choice of doctors or hospitals. Usually, you pay a yearly deductible and part of the cost of a visit (called a copayment).

Many health care professionals expect you to pay the total fee at the time of the service. You must then apply to your insurance company to be reimbursed for the money you spent. You should ask whether your doctor or hospital accepts "assignment" of benefits—that is, whether they will wait for your insurance company to pay its share. Compared with the prepaid health plans, FFS creates additional paperwork and the possibility of having to pay all expenses up front. Another disadvantage is that preventive health care (mammogram, Pap smear, or well-baby checkup) is often not covered. The advantage of the FFS system is that you have greater freedom of choice among health care professionals and area hospitals.

More questions to ask

Recently, there has been significant criticism of HMOs, especially those that are "for-profit." As a consumer, you should ask a variety of questions before joining a particular medical insurance plan. Due to the higher costs of health care with diabetes, you should have the answers to all these questions before deciding which insurance plan is best for you and your family.

In addition, you may want to find out whether any types of incentives are involved in your doctor's salary. For example, does your doctor make additional income by withholding certain types of care, even if recommended by the ADA clinical practice guidelines? Are there doctor incentives for using less expensive medications, when clearly a more expensive one would be better (such as using a diuretic instead of an angiotensin converting enzyme inhibitor for the treatment of hypertension with proteinuria)? Some doctors may not answer these types of questions due to a conflict of interest, but such considerations may be part of your doctor's decision-making process. It is easy to see how potential problems could arise.

What guidelines are followed

Quality of health care is something we are just beginning to measure. New buzzwords in medicine include *health-outcome measurements*, *evidence-based medicine*, and *practice guidelines*. These terms show that the treatment of any condition should be based on good clinical research, benefit society, and be cost effective. An excellent example of evidence-based medicine is the diabetes management recommendations based on the DCCT discussed in Chapter 3. We know that intensive therapy of type I diabetes results in much less retinopathy, nephropathy, and neuropathy. All the ADA Clinical Practice Recommendations, posi-

Questions to Ask Your
Insurance Company Before Joining

Are diabetes self-management education programs covered?

Will I be allowed to see an endocrinologist if I need to or want to?

Will I have access to a dietitian and nurse educator?

Will insulin, syringes, and diabetes pills be covered?

Will blood glucose monitoring supplies be covered?

Will a yearly dilated eye examination by an eye doctor be covered?

Will yearly urine tests for microalbumin be covered?

Are insulin pumps covered (or will pump supplies for my insulin pump be covered)?

Will I be allowed to see a podiatrist, and will there be coverage for my orthotics?

Will I have access to a mental health specialist, such as a medical social worker or psychologist?

Will I have access to an obstetrician experienced in pregnancies of women with diabetes and an endocrinologist during my pregnancy?

Are treatments for erectile dysfunction covered?

tion statements, and consensus statements covered in Chapter 1 are also examples of how research is translated into the daily practice of medicine.

If your provider is using practice guidelines for diabetes that are different from the ADA Clinical Practice Recommendations, you should ask why. Make sure that all of the current guidelines (for blood pressure, cholesterol levels, measurement of urine microalbumin, and so forth) are being followed.

There are ways to measure quality other than asking whether practice guidelines are being followed. How you and your doctor achieve your good health is also important. In the box, "Factors Necessary to Achieve Quality Health Care," you'll find other measures of health-care quality.

Accreditation of health plan

Just as doctors earn board certification, health plans now can become accredited. An independent agency known as the National Committee on Quality Assurance (NCQA) was formed to monitor both health-plan and doctor-group performance. The NCQA can be thought of as an employer and consumer advocate agency. It measures how well a health plan monitors the care its doctors give and, if the care is not adequate, the steps that are taken to improve it. Members' rights and satisfaction are also reviewed before accreditation.

Currently, there are more than 60 measures of quality used by the NCQA. They are regularly reviewed and updated. Unfortunately, there are no specific indicators by the NCQA for monitoring diabetes at this time. The focus of the NCQA is disease prevention, so it monitors things such as childhood immunizations and the number of people who receive Pap smears or cholesterol testing. Because prevention of disease is such an important part of the ADA Clinical Practice Recommendations, they would be ideal for health plans and their providers to follow.

To find out whether your health plan is NCQA accredited, you may call (202) 955-3500. The list of accredited plans may also be accessed via the World Wide Web at http://www.ncqa.org/. If your plan is not accredited, you should ask why and when it will become accredited.

Hopefully, insurance plans will incorporate ADA clinical practice guidelines into their care plans. Physician groups such as those in a staff-model HMO or within a clinic are beginning to develop these types of practice guidelines, noting treatment goals and providing specific ways to achieve these targets. Once the results of these experiments are published, including the information about the

---

Factors Necessary to Achieve Quality Health Care

- Achieves the best possible outcomes for you
- Helps you function to the best of your ability given your condition
- Sees you as often as meets your needs
- Is culturally and linguistically appropriate for you
- Involves your entire family, if necessary
- Is accessible and efficient
- Is provided in the most appropriate setting
- Is the least restrictive on your preferences
- Meets the most up-to-date professional standards of care
- Allows you to actively participate in clinical decisions
- Is a continuous and coordinated effort by a skilled health care team
- Is provided in a manner that respects you as a person
- Promotes health, and practices disease prevention

From Cafferky ME: *Managed Care & You: The Consumer Guide to Managing Your Health Care.* New York, McGraw-Hill, 1995.

---

cost and benefit (including cost savings) of this type of systematic diabetes treatment, this type of management will probably become available for most people with diabetes.

Appendix 1

Drugs Used for the Treatment of Diabetes

Insulin (based on information from manufacturers; duration and peak may differ among individuals).

INSULINS

SHORT ACTING	Onset	Peak	Duration
Humalog (Lilly)	15 min	1 hr	3.5–4.5 hrs
Humulin R (Lilly)	30 min	2–4 hrs	6–8 hrs
Velosulin BR (Novo Nordisk)	30 min	1–3 hrs	8 hrs
Novolin R (Novo Nordisk)	30 min	2.5–5 hr	6–8 hrs

INTERMEDIATE ACTING			
	Onset	Peak	Duration
Humulin L (Lilly)	1–3 hrs	6–12 hrs	18–24 hrs

INTERMEDIATE ACTING—cont'd

	Onset	Peak	Duration
Humulin NPH (Lilly)	1–2 hrs	6–12 hrs	18–24 hrs
Novolin L (Novo Nordisk)	2.5 hrs	7–15 hrs	22 hrs
NovolinN (Novo Nordisk)	1.5 hrs	4–12 hrs	24 hrs

LONG ACTING

	Onset	Peak	Duration
Humulin U (Lilly)	4–6 hrs	8–20 hrs	24–28 hrs

PREMIXED

	Onset	Peak	Duration
Humulin 70/30 (Lilly)	30 min	2–12 hrs	18–24 hrs
Humulin 50/50 (Lilly)	30 min	2–12 hrs	16–24 hrs
Novolin 70/30 (Novo Nordisk)	30 min	2–12 hrs	24 hrs

ORAL MEDICATIONS

SULFONYLUREAS	Daily Dose	Frequency (doses/day)
Tolbutamide Orinase	500–3000 mg	1–3
Chlorpropamide Diabinase	100–500 mg	1
Tolazamide Tolinase	100–1000 mg	1–2

ORAL MEDICATIONS—cont'd

SULFONYLUREAS	Daily Dose	Frequency (doses/day)
Glipizide Glucotrol	2.5–40 mg	1–2
Glipizide-GITS Glucotrol XL	5–20 mg	1
Glyburide Diabeta Micronase Glyburide, micronized form	1.25–20 mg	1–2
Glynase Biguanid Metformin	1.5–12 mg	1–2
Glucophage	1–2.5 grams	2–3

α-GLUCOSIDASE INHIBITOR	Daily Dose	Frequency (doses/day)
Acarbose Precose	50–100 mg	3

Appendix 2

Diabetes-Related World Wide Web Sites

There are now dozens of sites on the World Wide Web (WWW) devoted to diabetes and related topics. The following is a list of several sites you may want to visit first:

1. **http://www.diabetes.org/**
   This is the ADA home page. An excellent place to get started, because it provides much up-to-date information including stories about new research; a calendar of events, a list of books and journals; and links to the state affiliates.
2. **http://www.castleweb.com/%7Emonitor/**
   Diabetes Monitor; "monitoring diabetes everywhere in cyberspace."
3. **http://www.hsc.missouri.edu/modiabetes. index.html**
   Sponsored by the ADA Missouri Affiliate, the Missouri Department of Health Diabetes Control Program, and the University of Missouri Columbia Health Science Center, this site is a superb resource and includes a copy of the ADA Standards of Care.

4. http://www.noah.cuny.edu/diabetes.html
   Ask NOAH About Diabetes; an excellent
   overview of diabetes, providing both English and
   Spanish sites.
5. http://www.yahoo.com/Health/Diseases_
   and_conditions/diabetes/
   Yahoo's Diabetes Links; an excellent gateway to
   other diabetes links.
6. http://www.cdc.gov/nccdphp/ddt/ddthome. html
   Centers for Disease Control Diabetes Home Page;
   an excellent resource.
7. http://www.castleweb.com/diabetes/ index.htlm
   Children with Diabetes; "The on-line magazine for
   kids, families, and adults with juvenile diabetes."
8. http://www.findcure.org/%7Ediabetes/
   ADA Oregon Affiliate Home Page; interesting
   reading even if you don't live in Oregon.
9. http://www.ncqa.org/
   National Committee on Quality Assurance Home
   Page; this organization monitors both health-plan
   and physician-group performance and can be used
   when choosing among health plans, including
   HMOs.

Glossary

albuminuria—when albumin, a type of protein, appears in the urine.

atherosclerosis—when an artery is blocked by plaque, a collection of fat, complex carbohydrates, and blood protein.

cardiovascular disease—any disease of the heart or circulatory system; coronary artery disease can result in a heart attack, cerebral vascular disease can result in a stroke, and peripheral vascular disease can result in gangrene of the feet and amputation.

cholesterol—fat necessary for making cell membranes and certain hormones; it is in food from animal products or produced by the body.

claudication—pain in the legs and feet due to a decrease in blood flow from peripheral vascular disease; usually, the pain is worse with exercise and better with rest.

diabetologist—endocrinologist who specializes in the treatment of diabetes.

endocrine glands—places in the body where hormones are made.

endocrinologist—doctor who specializes in diseases of the endocrine system (all of the glands that make hormones).

epinephrine—also called adrenaline, this hormone comes from the adrenal gland; raises blood pressure and blood glucose, helping to keep blood glucose levels normal when too much insulin is available.

gastroparesis—effect of autonomic neuropathy in which food is not moved from the stomach to the rest of the intestine normally; can result in symptoms of feeling full after a small amount of food, bloating, nausea, and vomiting; a "mismatching" of food absorption and injected insulin can result in after-meal hypoglycemia.

genitourinary system—the genital and urinary organs: kidney, ureter, bladder, urethra, prostate, vagina, ovaries, testes, and penis.

gestational diabetes—diabetes which occurs only during pregnancy, and goes away afterwards; indicates an increased risk of developing type II.

glucagon—a hormone secreted by the pancreas, it raises blood glucose; it can be injected to treat hypoglycemia.

glycated hemoglobin—also called glycosylated hemoglobin; a measure of blood glucose control for the previous 12–16 weeks.

glycosuria—appearance of glucose in the urine.

hormones—substances made in the body and transported through the blood to cause an action at another part of the body.

hyperglycemia—higher-than-normal blood glucose level; symptoms are frequent urination, thirst, blurry vision, and often weight loss.

hypertension—high blood pressure.

hypoglycemia—low blood glucose level caused by too much insulin (or sulfonylurea), not enough food, or too much exercise; symptoms are hunger, nervousness, profuse sweating, tremor, or even seizures or coma.

hypothyroidism—low thyroid hormone levels, a common condition in the general population and even more common with type I diabetes; symptoms are fatigue, cold intolerance, constipation, dry skin, and coarse hair.

insulin-dependent diabetes mellitus—type I diabetes; accounts for only about 10% of all people with diabetes; without insulin, patients will develop ketoacidosis and die; people are usually not obese and develop diabetes during childhood or adolescence.

insulin resistance—problem in type II diabetes or with obesity; insulin doesn't work as it should so it takes more to lower blood glucose.

intensive diabetes therapy—system of diabetes management including daily self-monitoring of blood glucose, individualized blood glucose goals, frequent contact with health care team, and multiple daily insulin injections or insulin pump therapy.

ketoacidosis—life-threatening emergency; not enough insulin causes fat breakdown and ketone formation; ketones are acids that in large quantities, can be extremely dangerous; this condition is usually seen with very high blood glucose levels and severe dehydration.

ketone—by-product of fat breakdown when not enough insulin is present.

ketonuria—appearance of ketones in the urine.

microalbuminuria—tiny amounts of albumin, a type of protein in the urine; first sign of diabetic kidney disease and signals increased risk for heart attack.

microvascular—referring to small blood vessels, such as those seen in the kidney and retina.

non-insulin-dependent diabetes mellitus—type II diabetes; accounts for 90% of cases of diabetes; insulin is not required for survival; patients are usually obese and develop diabetes after age 40.

orthostatic hypotension—low blood pressure on standing; can occur from dehydration due to high blood glucose levels or from autonomic neuropathy.

osteomyelitis—bone infection; can lead to amputation when it occurs in the feet.

podiatrist—health care provider specializing in diseases of the feet.

proteinuria—protein in the urine; first sign of diabetic kidney disease and a factor for heart attack.

retina—multilayered structure lining back wall of the eye.

retinopathy (diabetic)—condition that, in its mild form (nonproliferative), is characterized by small bleeds and protein deposits and may cause visual loss (macular edema); severe form (proliferative) characterized by growth of new blood vessels and greater risk of loss of vision.

severe hypoglycemia—low blood glucose requiring the assistance of another person for treatment.

SMBG—self-monitoring of blood glucose.

sulfonylurea—oral medication that lowers blood glucose levels in type II diabetes; stimulates insulin secretion, so hypoglycemia is possible.

triglycerides—major kind of fat in foods; these particles are also created by our bodies to store excess calories to provide energy in the future.

urinary incontinence—inability to control passing of urine.

Index